MASTER MENOPAUSE

Overcome Fear of losing your identity, Break Free from isolation, Navigate the hormonal changes, and Reclaim Control of your body and life

EVA HARMONY

SquatchCo LLC

Copyright © 2024 Eva Harmony.

All rights reserved. No part of this publication may be reproduced, distributed, or transmitted in any form or by any means, including photocopying, recording, or other electronic or mechanical methods, without the prior written permission of the publisher or author, except in the case of brief quotations embodied in critical reviews and certain other noncommercial uses permitted by copyright law.

ISBN: 979-8-9920524-0-4

Published by SquatchCo LLC

Eugene, Oregon, USA

Disclaimer Notice:

Please note that the information contained within this document is for educational and entertainment purposes only. Every effort has been made to present accurate, up-to-date, and reliable, complete information. No warranties of any kind are declared or implied. Readers acknowledge that the author is not engaging in the rendering of legal, financial, medical or professional advice. The content within this book has been derived from various sources. **Please consult a licensed professional before attempting any techniques outlined in this book.**

By reading this, the reader agrees that under no circumstances is the author or publisher responsible for any losses, direct or indirect, which are incurred as a result of the use of the information contained within this document, including, but not limited to, — errors, omissions, or inaccuracies.

CONTENTS

Introduction	vii
1. Demystifying Menopause	1
2. Identifying Symptoms, Their Impact, and Relief Strategies	15
3. Emotional Well-being During Menopause	25
4. Relationships and Intimacy	39
5. Diet and Nutrition	49
6. Exercise and Physical Health	61
7. Understanding Hormone Replacement Therapy (HRT)	73
8. Natural & Alternative Remedies and Complementary Therapies	83
9. Self-Care and Empowerment	91
10. Moving Forward with Confidence	103
Conclusion	117
References	119

INTRODUCTION

Whether you're approaching menopause, in the midst of it, or simply curious about what lies ahead, this book is more than just a guide-it's your trusted ally. It's natural to feel overwhelmed by the changes your body and mind are undergoing, but together, we can navigate this transition with knowledge and confidence.

Understanding menopause goes beyond grappling with symptoms; it's about redefining a significant part of your life in a way that embraces change with knowledge, support, and empowerment. As you move through the pages of this book, remember that each piece of information is a stepping stone toward mastering your menopause transition, tailored to respect your unique experience and personal journey.

Why This Book? Menopause is more than just a biological process; it's a complex experience that impacts every aspect of your life. In *Master Menopause*, my aim is to demystify the physical, emotional, and social effects of menopause. By sharing valuable knowledge, personal stories, and practical advice, I hope to empower you to manage these changes proactively.

Inclusivity is a cornerstone of this book. It is carefully crafted for all women, including those dealing with health conditions like breast cancer or autoimmune diseases that might uniquely shape their menopausal experience. Everyone's story is important, and every experience deserves to be heard and understood.

Master Menopause is structured to guide you through understanding menopause, managing symptoms, enhancing emotional well-being, making lifestyle adjustments, and exploring treatments beyond the traditional scope. This journey will take you from uncertainty to mastery, from feeling out of control to reclaiming your body and life.

Our holistic approach addresses not only the physical symptoms but also the emotional, psychological, and social dynamics of menopause. This comprehensive viewpoint equips you to handle not just the hot flashes but also any feelings of isolation or shifts in identity.

Expect a book free from extreme diets, medical jargon, and outdated stereotypes. Instead, you'll find engaging, thoughtful content that not only respects your intelligence but also reflects the diverse experiences of menopause because your journey is unique and deserves to be understood.

My inspiration for writing this book stems from witnessing the transformative journeys of many remarkable women, including close friends and family. Their strength and vulnerability in facing menopause motivated me to create a resource that can support others in similar situations.

Did you know that nearly 80 percent of women experience menopausal symptoms, yet many feel unprepared to deal with these changes? This gap between experience and knowledge is what *Master Menopause* aims to bridge. Let's challenge misconceptions and reveal the true nature of menopause so you can feel informed and empowered.

Join me on this empowering journey. Let's explore, learn, and grow together through the pages of this book. Menopause is more than an end to fertility; it is a beginning to a new and potentially fulfilling phase of life. We can navigate it together with courage, support, and heart.

DEMYSTIFYING MENOPAUSE

In a world brimming with information and advice, the true essence of menopause often remains shrouded in mystery and misconceptions. As you stand at the threshold of what might seem like an uncertain phase, this chapter will illuminate the path by providing a clear understanding of what menopause entails. Not merely a medical condition to be managed, menopause is a significant life transition that encompasses biological, emotional, and societal dimensions. Here, you will find facts and narratives that resonate with your experiences and knowledge, empowering you to navigate menopause confidently and positively.

THE MENOPAUSE TRANSITION: MORE THAN JUST AN END TO PERIODS

Menopause is often associated simply with the end of monthly periods, but it is much more than just that. It is a natural biological process that marks the end of reproductive fertility, not just a single event. This transition typically spans several years, often beginning in your 40s and stretching into your 50s and sometimes beyond. It is a gradual process that involves a series of changes, not only in your reproductive hormones but across your entire body systems, influencing your physical health, emotional well-being, and social interactions.

The Phases of Menopause

Understanding the phases of menopause can significantly demystify the experience and help you anticipate and manage changes more effectively. The transition into menopause is typically divided into three key phases: perimenopause, menopause, and postmenopause.

> **Perimenopause:** This phase often begins several years before menopause, when the ovaries gradually produce less estrogen. It's during perimenopause that many women experience the most acute symptoms of the transition, such as irregular periods, hot flashes, sleep disturbances, and mood swings. It's a time of significant hormonal fluctuation that can feel like a rollercoaster for many.
> **Menopause:** This phase is defined as twelve consecutive months without a menstrual period. By this time, the ovaries have significantly reduced the production of hormones like estrogen and progesterone. While some symptoms may persist, this phase often brings a new set of adjustments as your body adapts to lower levels of reproductive hormones.
> **Postmenopause:** The years following menopause can bring a sense of relief to many as the intense symptoms of perimenopause begin to wane. However, postmenopause can also bring challenges, including increased risks of conditions like osteoporosis and heart disease due to ongoing lower estrogen levels.

Symptom Spectrum

Menopausal symptoms vary widely among women, so personal stories are crucial for understanding the full spectrum of potential experiences. While one woman might suffer severe hot flashes and night sweats, another might notice mood swings or memory lapses as more pronounced symptoms. Still others might experience vaginal dryness, changes in libido, or joint pains. This variability underscores the need for a personalized approach to managing menopause, as no single approach works for everyone.

Cultural Recognition and Misconceptions

Menopause has been enveloped in silence and, occasionally, stigma. This lack of open dialogue can lead to misconceptions and myths about menopause that are pervasive and damaging. In some cultures, menopause is viewed negatively as a signal of aging and decline, contributing to stereotypes that marginalize older women. Fortunately, more progressive narratives are emerging that recognize menopause as a phase of empowerment, wisdom, and liberation. By challenging the negative stereotypes and embracing a more informed, positive perspective, we can foster a respectful and appreciative view of menopause.

HORMONES IN FLUX: WHY YOUR BODY FEELS DIFFERENT

The fluctuations in your hormone levels during menopause are more than just numbers on a medical chart; they are central to your bodily experiences during this transition. The decline in estrogen and progesterone ripples across your entire body, influencing everything from temperature regulation to cardiovascular health.

Hormonal Changes Explained

Estrogen and progesterone, the primary female reproductive hormones, play pivotal roles beyond fertility. Estrogen influences over 400 functions in your body, including maintaining body temperature, preserving bone density, and regulating cholesterol levels in the blood. As you approach menopause, the ovaries gradually reduce hormone production, leading to decreased levels that affect these vital functions. This reduction is more of a turbulent descent than a steady decline, which explains the sudden onset of hot flashes and unpredictable mood swings.

Physical Effects of Hormonal Shifts

Hot flashes, night sweats, and mood swings—the symptoms most commonly associated with menopause—are directly tied to the hormonal upheaval occurring in your body. Hot flashes result from unstable temperature regulation; your body suddenly feels overheated, even when there is no physical need to cool down. Sleep disturbances arise from the decrease in progesterone, which has soothing properties that help promote sleep and hot flashes. Mood swings can be attributed to the direct influence of estrogen on neurotransmitters in the brain, such as serotonin and dopamine, which affect mood regulation. These symptoms are your body's response to the new hormonal environment it finds itself in.

Long-Term Health Implications

While the immediate symptoms of menopause are challenging, the long-term health implications require equal attention. The decline in estrogen levels is linked to an increase in the risk of osteoporosis and heart disease. Estrogen helps absorb calcium and other minerals into the bones—its decline can mean diminished bone density and greater susceptibility to fractures. Estrogen also affects the flexibility of the arterial walls and helps to maintain healthy cholesterol levels. Thus, its protective effects on the heart are lessened during menopause, increasing the risk of cardiovascular disease.

Navigating Hormonal Flux

Managing these symptoms and risks effectively involves a combination of lifestyle adjustments, medical interventions, and, crucially, understanding your body's new normal. Diet and exercise become even more essential. A diet rich in calcium and vitamin D can help mitigate the loss of bone density, while regular physical activity, particularly weight-bearing exercises, can help maintain bone strength. For heart health, a diet low in saturated fats and high in fiber can help manage cholesterol levels, complemented by cardiovascular exercises to keep the heart strong. Understanding and anticipating hormonal changes will help you manage your health proactively as you navigate this phase.

MENOPAUSE ACROSS CULTURES: A GLOBAL PERSPECTIVE

The menopause experience varies significantly across different cultures and societies. These variations are not just minor differences in symptoms but profound divergences in how menopause is perceived, experienced, and supported. Understanding these differences enriches our global perspective and allows us to extract valuable lessons from societies that may have a more holistic or supportive approach to this significant life transition.

Cultural Attitudes

Across the globe, cultural attitudes toward menopause range from stigmatizing to celebratory. Western societies tend to treat menopause as a medical issue, emphasizing the loss of fertility and youth. This perspective often generates a sense of dread or stigma around menopause. In contrast, indigenous cultures in which women are valued for their wisdom and experience, not merely their fertility, perceive menopause as a time of liberation and respect. For example, among the Bantu-speaking groups in Africa, menopausal women often gain social status and are valued as decision-makers within their communities. This more positive value to society can significantly alter a woman's menopause experience, even transforming it into a phase to look forward to.

Community Support

The role of community, healthcare, and family in supporting menopausal women varies widely. In Japan, for instance, menopause (known as "konenki") is openly discussed, and there is substantial community and family support, which helps women cope better with the symptoms and changes. The Japanese healthcare system also tends to adopt a more integrative approach to menopause management, combining conventional medicine with traditional remedies and practices. On the other hand, in some Middle Eastern cultures, open dialogue about menopause is often discouraged, and the resulting lack of support from family or healthcare systems can lead to feelings of isolation during menopause. The disparity underscores the need for education and global dialogue about menopause, aiming to foster supportive environments where women feel supported and understood regardless of their geographic or cultural location.

Cultural Insights

There are profound lessons to be learned from cultures that embrace a more positive and holistic approach to menopause. In some Native American tribes, menopause is considered a sacred time when a woman enters the "Wise Woman' phase. This cultural reverence can significantly improve and positively affect a woman's self-esteem and mental health. Adopting such perspectives could help shift the narrative around menopause in cultures where it is viewed negatively. The use of specific natural remedies and lifestyle adjustments in these cultures, which focus on holistic well-being rather than just treating symptoms, can offer alternative approaches that might be integrated into more conventional treatment plans. These practices broaden the treatment landscape and emphasize the importance of viewing menopause as a natural life stage rather than a medical problem to be fixed.

THE SCIENCE BEHIND SYMPTOMS: WHAT'S NORMAL AND WHAT'S NOT

Navigating menopause can often feel like trying to find your way through a dense fog—symptoms can appear out of nowhere and might even alarm you with their intensity or strangeness. Understanding which symptoms are typical of menopause and which might indicate other health issues is crucial for your peace of mind and for managing your health proactively during this transition. This clarity begins with a detailed exploration of the biological symptoms, providing a foundation for building knowledge.

Common vs. Uncommon Symptoms

The hallmark symptoms of menopause—hot flashes, night sweats, irregular periods, and mood swings—are experienced by a significant number of women and are generally no cause for alarm. However, the intensity and combination of these symptoms vary widely. Most women will experience mild to moderate hot flashes, but for some, severe hot flashes that negatively affect their quality of life are the norm. Similarly, mild mood swings that slightly affect your emotional well-being are common. Yet, if you find yourself experiencing severe depression or anxiety, this is a sign that you might need to seek additional help. Other less common but concerning symptoms might include significant weight loss, extreme fatigue, or postmenopausal bleeding, which are reasons to consult a healthcare provider.

Biological Basis of Symptoms

Menopause symptoms are closely linked to the hormonal changes in your body. Estrogen and progesterone, the primary hormones regulating the menstrual cycle, also influence a variety of bodily functions, including temperature regulation, mood, metabolism, and bone density. As you transition into menopause, fluctuating hormone levels can lead to a variety of symptoms. Hot flashes and night sweats, for example, are directly related to how declining estrogen levels affect the hypothalamus, the part of your brain that regulates body temperature. Mood swings correlate with how these hormonal changes impact neurotransmitter activity in your brain, affecting how you feel and react to situations.

The decrease in estrogen that comes with menopause can also affect the mucous membranes, leading to dryness, which is why vaginal dryness and changes in skin texture are also common during this time. By understanding the biological roots of these symptoms, you can better grasp why certain treatments or lifestyle changes — like hormone replacement therapy for severe hot flashes or vaginal lubricants for dryness— are recommended.

When to Seek Help

Recognizing the difference between typical symptoms and more severe issues is crucial for effective management. Consult a healthcare provider if you experience symptoms that severely impact your quality of life, are unusual, or don't respond to standard management strategies. For example, if sleep disturbances are causing persistent insomnia that affects your daily functioning or if mood swings evolve into prolonged depression or anxiety, professional guidance can help you manage these effectively.

A healthcare provider should immediately evaluate any post-menopausal bleeding as this could indicate other medical conditions, including, but not limited to, endometrial hyperplasia or even cancer. Staying informed about these symptoms and understanding when they might signal something more serious is crucial for taking action.

EARLY ONSET AND PREMATURE MENOPAUSE: SPECIAL CONSIDERATIONS

Understanding the nuances between early onset and premature menopause is crucial. Early-onset menopause occurs between the ages of 40 and 45. Premature menopause, on the other hand, happens before the age of 40. Both conditions are considered variations of early menopause but differ in severity and impact. Recognizing these differences helps in managing expectations and tailoring interventions.

Causes of early and premature menopause include genetic, surgical, and environmental factors. Some women inherit a tendency for earlier menopause from their mothers or grandmothers, indicating a family pattern. Surgical interventions, such as hysterectomy or any surgery that impacts the ovaries, can trigger menopause if the ovaries are removed or if their blood supply is compromised. Environmental factors like smoking and exposure to certain chemicals and toxins can disrupt hormonal balance and are sometimes linked to earlier menopause. Autoimmune diseases, where the body mistakenly attacks its tissues, can affect the ovaries and lead to early menopause. Understanding these causes is crucial for recognizing risks and exploring preventive measures.

Entering menopause early affects more than just menstruation. Fertility takes a direct hit. Women who enter menopause early often face unexpected challenges in conceiving naturally, which can be emotionally distressing, especially if they have plans for children later in life. Early loss of estrogen increases the risk of osteoporosis, heart disease, and even certain types of dementia. The emotional toll and these health risks necessitate a supportive approach that addresses physical and psychological needs.

Support and treatment options for women experiencing early or premature menopause need to be comprehensive. Hormone replacement therapy (HRT) is commonly recommended to counter the deficiency of estrogen and to mitigate the risks associated with its early loss. However, the decision to start HRT should be made after a thorough discussion with a healthcare provider, considering the potential benefits and risks. Support groups and counseling can play pivotal roles in helping women cope with the emotional aspects of premature menopause. These groups provide a platform for sharing experiences and offer solace in knowing one is not alone in this journey. Lifestyle changes, such as adopting a diet rich in calcium and vitamin D, practicing regular weight-bearing exercise, and smoking cessation, are also crucial in managing health risks associated with early menopause.

By understanding the underlying causes of early onset and premature menopause, recognizing the broader implications, and exploring comprehensive treatment and support systems, women can better manage this unexpected transition.

MENOPAUSE ACROSS CULTURES: A GLOBAL PERSPECTIVE

Menopause, a universal biological milestone, is perceived and experienced through a diverse cultural lens around the globe. These perceptions heavily influence the individual's experience and the societal support structures for women navigating this transition. Understanding these varied landscapes offers invaluable insights into how different societies embrace or stigmatize menopause, shaping the well-being of women worldwide.

Cultural Attitudes

Cultural attitudes profoundly impact how women perceive and handle this change. In many Western societies, menopause is often medicalized and treated as a disorder, which can foster feelings of inadequacy or anxiety among women. In contrast, in some Asian cultures, menopause is viewed as a natural transition that signifies wisdom and maturity. In Japan, this phase is called "konenki" and is seen as a time for personal growth and renewal. Such cultural affirmation can significantly alleviate the psychological burden of menopause, providing a more supportive environment for women.

Indigenous cultures of North and South America often celebrate menopause as a rite of passage conferring social privileges and respect. Women in these cultures frequently have a more positive menopause experience, suggesting a strong link between cultural attitudes and the manifestation of menopausal symptoms. These examples highlight the powerful influence of societal norms and values on the health and well-being of women during menopause. Shifting the narrative to one of empowerment and respect can transform the menopausal experience for many women across different societies.

Societal Support Systems

The role of societal support systems in managing menopause is as varied as the cultures themselves. In Scandinavia, robust healthcare support for women—including menopause clinics and educational programs—helps women manage symptoms effectively. Open discussions about menopause in these societies help women feel more prepared and supported during this transition.

Conversely, in parts of the Middle East and Africa, a lack of open dialogue about menopause often results in minimal institutional support, leaving women to navigate this phase, in some cases without any guidance or assistance. Family plays a crucial role in providing the primary support network in these regions. Without broader community and healthcare support, women's options for managing symptoms and accessing treatment are severely limited. This disparity highlights the need for comprehensive support systems that include healthcare, education, and community awareness to create a supportive environment for menopausal women.

Learning from Others

Cultures with a holistic approach to menopause offer valuable lessons. For instance, Chinese herbal remedies and traditional medicine provide alternative strategies for managing symptoms that are less reliant on hormone replacement therapies prevalent in Western medicine. These practices broaden the spectrum of available treatments and inspire a more natural approach to managing health transitions.

Community involvement in cultures where menopause is openly discussed and celebrated can be a model for creating support networks elsewhere. Such communities often experience lower rates of depression and isolation among menopausal women, highlighting the importance of social support and acceptance in promoting mental health and well-being during menopause.

Promoting a Global Dialogue

The diverse global experiences of menopause provide a rich tapestry of knowledge that can be shared across cultural boundaries. Promoting a global dialogue about menopause can help dispel myths and misconceptions, spread effective practices, and foster a more supportive and informed global community. Such dialogue enhances awareness and encourages adapting best practices that can be customized to fit different cultural contexts.

Engaging in this conversation requires openness and respect for cultural diversity. We must recognize that each culture has unique insights and practices that contribute to a comprehensive understanding of menopause. By embracing this dialogue, we can work toward a world where menopause is not feared but managed with dignity and support, allowing every woman to transition through this phase of life with confidence.

BEYOND BIOLOGY: THE SOCIAL DIMENSIONS OF MENOPAUSE

The portrayal of menopause in popular culture strongly influences how women perceive and experience this life stage. Often depicted with humor or pity, menopause in films, television, and various media platforms frequently focuses on the more challenging symptoms like hot flashes and mood swings. The positive aspects of menopause are often overlooked, leading to a skewed perception of it as a period of decline rather than a phase of liberation and potential growth. This portrayal not only perpetuates stereotypes that isolate women going through menopause but also can make them feel that their experiences are too trivial or embarrassing to discuss openly.

The media can better represent menopause experiences by showcasing both the challenges and triumphs. A balanced portrayal is crucial in normalizing this natural life transition. Imagine a TV series featuring a middle-aged protagonist embracing new life challenges or a documentary exploring menopause from scientific and holistic perspectives. These portrayals could encourage open dialogue and reduce the stigma associated with menopause.

The Role of Community and Conversation

Creating a supportive community through open discussions about menopause is essential for changing perceptions and providing support. The silence around menopause can lead to misinformation and isolation. By fostering environments where women feel safe and supported in sharing their experiences, we can build a collective wisdom that empowers all women to navigate menopause more confidently.

Online and offline communities play a pivotal role in this aspect. Online forums and social media groups can offer spaces where women from diverse backgrounds share advice, stories, and support. Local community centers, healthcare facilities, and even informal coffee meetings can have vital discussions about menopause. These gatherings provide important information and help to forge connections among women at similar life stages, which is invaluable in breaking the isolation often associated with menopause.

The role of healthcare providers in these conversations cannot be overstated. When doctors, nurses, and other health professionals are equipped to initiate discussions about menopause openly and knowledgeably, it helps to normalize the conversation, integrating it into routine health care. This approach ensures that women receive comprehensive information and support tailored to their needs.

Challenging the Stigma

Challenging negative perceptions of menopause requires proactive efforts from individuals and communities alike. Education is one effective strategy—promoting factual, positive information about menopause. This might involve organizing community talks, distributing informative pamphlets, or even personal blogs and articles that tackle menopause from a fresh perspective.

Advocacy is another powerful approach. By advocating for better menopausal care and support in workplaces and institutions, we can drive changes that acknowledge and accommodate the needs of menopausal women. This includes advocating for policies like flexible work hours or thermal comfort in workplaces, which can make a significant difference for those experiencing menopausal symptoms.

On a personal level, open discussions with friends, family, and colleagues can be transformative. Sharing your own experiences or supporting a friend not only provides immediate comfort but also further changes the narrative around menopause from one of embarrassment or anxiety to one of acceptance and normalcy.

Transforming how menopause is perceived and experienced means improving the lives of individual women—we are reshaping societal norms and creating a legacy of respect, support, and empowerment for future generations. By breaking down barriers and stigma, we create a society that embraces all stages of a woman's life with compassion and respect, recognizing the strength and wisdom that come with each passing year.

Menopause is a natural phase of life that carries challenges and growth opportunities. By embracing knowledge, fostering open conversations, and building supportive communities, we can reshape the narrative around menopause. This chapter has addressed the need to recognize each woman's unique experiences and advocate for respectful treatment and understanding. As we continue to share our stories and learn from diverse cultural perspectives, we can create a more compassionate world where menopause is celebrated as a transformative journey, empowering women to embrace this life transition with confidence and dignity.

IDENTIFYING SYMPTOMS, THEIR IMPACT, AND RELIEF STRATEGIES

As you navigate menopause, understanding the symptoms you encounter is not just about knowing what they are but understanding why they occur and how to manage them effectively. This chapter delves into some of the most common yet challenging menopause symptoms—hot flashes and night sweats. These symptoms are not merely physical nuisances but signals that your body needs attention and care. Here, you will learn how to interpret these signals and respond to them with strategies that bring comfort and relief, integrating natural remedies, lifestyle adjustments, and stress management techniques into your daily life.

HOT FLASHES AND NIGHT SWEATS: COOLING DOWN NATURALLY

Menopause's notorious symptoms—hot flashes and night sweats—can make you feel like your body's thermostat has gone haywire, overwhelming you with heat at the most inconvenient times. Medically known as vasomotor symptoms, these affect about 75% of menopausal women and are among the most common complaints for seeking medical advice during this transition. But what triggers these intense episodes? The root cause is how fluctuating estrogen levels affect your body's internal temperature regulation. Estrogen influences the hypothalamus, the part of your brain that controls body temperature. As menopause progresses and estrogen levels drop, the hypothalamus mistakenly senses that your body is overheating. This miscommunication triggers your body to disperse the supposed excess heat, resulting in the sudden warmth, sweating, and even shivering associated with hot flashes and night sweats.

Triggers for these episodes can vary widely among women. Understanding these triggers is the first step toward managing them and reducing the frequency and intensity of unpleasant episodes.

Lifestyle Adjustments

Modifying your lifestyle can radically reduce hot flashes and night sweats. Simple changes to your diet, clothing, and environmental changes can be your first line of defense. Wearing layers of light, breathable fabrics can help manage the heat during a hot flash, allowing you to adjust your temperature by removing layers as needed. Keeping your sleeping and living environments cool and well-ventilated can also provide significant relief. Consider using a fan in your bedroom at night and lowering the thermostat slightly to maintain a cooler overall temperature.

Diet also plays a crucial role. Certain foods and drinks can trigger or worsen hot flashes and night sweats. Reducing your intake of spicy foods, caffeine, and alcohol can help manage these symptoms more effectively. Instead, focus on incorporating phytoestrogen-rich foods, such as soybeans, flaxseeds, and whole grains, into your diet. Phytoestrogens are plant-derived compounds that can mimic the effects of estrogen in the body, potentially helping to stabilize the fluctuations that contribute to hot flashes and night sweats.

Natural Remedies

In addition to lifestyle changes, certain natural supplements and herbs can help manage hot flashes and night sweats. Black cohosh, for example, is one of the most well-researched herbs for menopausal symptoms. It is noted to have estrogen-like effects on the body, which may help stabilize temperature regulation. Other herbs, such as red clover, evening primrose oil, and sage, have also been used to alleviate vasomotor symptoms. Always consult a healthcare provider before starting any new supplement, as some herbs can interact with medications and may not be suitable for everyone.

Stress Management Techniques

Stress is a well-known trigger for hot flashes and night sweats, and managing your stress levels can go a long way in controlling these symptoms. Techniques such as yoga and meditation can help reduce stress and improve overall quality of life. Yoga combines physical postures, breathing exercises, and meditation to enhance your physical and mental health, making it particularly beneficial for menopausal women. Regular practice can help control your body's stress response and may reduce the frequency of hot flashes and night sweats.

Meditation—particularly mindfulness meditation—can also be a powerful tool. By training your mind to focus on the present moment and observe your thoughts and sensations without judgment, mindfulness helps reduce stress and promotes relaxation. Even a few minutes of daily meditation can make a significant difference in how you manage stress and experience menopausal symptoms.

Reflective Journal Prompt

Consider maintaining a menopause symptom journal. Regularly jot down the occurrence and intensity of your hot flashes and night sweats, noting what you were doing, eating, or feeling at the time. This practice can help you identify specific patterns and triggers, making it easier to manage your symptoms effectively. Reflect on how lifestyle adjustments, natural remedies, and stress management techniques affect your symptoms and what changes might further benefit your well-being.

MOOD SWINGS AND EMOTIONAL ROLLERCOASTERS: STABILIZING YOUR INNER CLIMATE

Navigating the emotional tide of menopause can sometimes feel like being adrift in a storm without an anchor. Fluctuating hormone levels trigger physical changes and deeply impact your emotions, leading to mood swings that might leave you feeling like you are out of control. Estrogen plays a key role in regulating the body's chemical messengers, or neurotransmitters such as serotonin and dopamine, which influence mood. As these hormone levels ebb and flow, so can your emotional state, sometimes leading to feelings of joy one moment and profound sadness or irritation the next. This volatility can be exhausting and confusing—both for you and your loved ones.

Understanding the connection between these hormonal changes and your emotions is the first step toward regaining stability. Recognizing that these feelings are a normal part of the menopause transition can help mitigate feelings of isolation or frustration. It's also essential to monitor these emotional changes closely, as they can sometimes indicate more serious conditions, such as depression or anxiety disorders, which may require professional intervention. Paying attention to your emotional health is as important as managing your physical health; both require attention and care.

Building resilience against these emotional upheavals involves cultivating a support system and employing strategies to enhance mental well-being. Mindful breathing or guided meditation can help anchor your thoughts and calm your mind. These practices guide you to live in the present moment and can provide a new perspective to handle emotions in healthier ways.

Therapy can be an invaluable resource. Speaking with a mental health professional helps you unpack the complexities of your feelings and provides strategies to cope with emotional instability. Cognitive-behavioral therapy (CBT) effectively alters unproductive thoughts and actions, improves emotional control, and creates coping mechanisms to tackle problems effectively.

Cultivating a support network of friends, family, and peers navigating menopause can provide emotional comfort and validation. Sharing stories and hearing how others cope with similar challenges can lessen your feelings of isolation and provide strategies for managing similar challenges. Similarly, regular social activities can boost your mood and give you a sense of normalcy amid the changes.

The role of nutrition in emotional health during menopause is often underestimated. The foods you eat can influence your brain's structure and function, affecting your mood and cognitive processes. For instance, omega-3 fatty acids found in fish, such as salmon and sardines, contribute to the structural stability of brain cells and are key to emotional health. Foods rich in vitamin B—such as leafy greens, whole grains, and legumes—are important for serotonin production, which can enhance mood and alleviate depression. On the other hand, consuming a high amount of refined sugars and processed foods can lead to fluctuations in blood sugar levels, potentially triggering mood swings.

SLEEP SOLUTIONS: RESTFUL NIGHTS WITHOUT MEDICATION

Sleep can become a recurring battle during menopause, transforming what should be a peaceful respite into hours of tossing and turning. Menopausal symptoms like hot flashes and anxiety are notorious for disrupting sleep patterns. A hot flash at night, often termed a night sweat, can jolt you awake with intense warmth, leaving your sleepwear and sheets uncomfortably damp. Anxiety—fueled by hormonal fluctuations—can keep your mind racing with worry or stress when you should be drifting off to sleep.

Understanding how these symptoms affect your sleep is crucial. Night sweats can disrupt your body's natural temperature regulation, making achieving and maintaining sleep's deep, restorative stages difficult. Anxiety, meanwhile, can trigger a cascade of stress hormones that keep the body in a state of heightened alertness, incompatible with the relaxation needed for sleep. These symptoms, whether experienced together or separately, lead to significant sleep deprivation. This will not only impact your physical health by increasing the risk of conditions such as heart disease and diabetes but will also affect your daily functioning and quality of life.

Developing a personalized approach to sleep hygiene is essential. Sleep hygiene includes the habits and practices that promote regular, restful sleep. Establish a bedtime routine to signal your body that it's time to wind down. Activities such as reading, taking a warm bath, or listening to calming music can help transition to a restful sleep state.

Creating a tranquil sleep environment is crucial for a good night's rest. Ensuring your bedroom is cool, quiet, and dark is essential, as these conditions support natural sleep processes. Use blackout curtains to block out light, a fan or air conditioner to maintain a cool temperature, and earplugs or a white noise machine to eliminate disruptive sounds. Investing in a quality mattress and pillows that provide comfortable support is also important for maximum relaxation.

Exploring alternative therapies like aromatherapy and sound therapy can provide relief from sleep disturbances without medication. Aromatherapy uses scents like lavender and chamomile to induce sleep, while sound therapy uses soothing sounds to create a tranquil environment that promotes sleep.

If you've tried improving your sleep habits and using alternative therapies but still experience sleep problems that impact your daily life, seeking professional help is vital. Consulting a healthcare provider can lead to a thorough evaluation and access to proven treatments like cognitive-behavioral therapy for insomnia (CBT-I). A healthcare provider should also investigate other potential causes of insomnia, such as sleep apnea or restless legs syndrome, to ensure you receive comprehensive care tailored to your needs.

By implementing helpful sleep hygiene practices, you can reclaim your nights and restore peace to your days.

NAVIGATING BRAIN FOG: CLEARING THE MENTAL MIST

Menopause brings many changes, and among the less discussed yet impactful are the cognitive shifts many women experience. The symptom, sometimes called "brain fog," can manifest as forgetfulness, difficulty concentrating, and trouble with word retrieval. These cognitive hiccups can be frustrating, affecting your professional performance, social interactions, and self-esteem. Recognizing that these changes are a normal part of menopause and not a reflection of your capabilities is key to managing them effectively.

Fluctuating hormone levels mainly cause brain fog. Estrogen—known to protect and enhance brain function—decreases during menopause, potentially affecting cognitive sharpness. This hormonal change can impact neurotransmitter function and brain cell activity, resulting in reduced clarity or brain fog. It's important to recognize these symptoms for personal understanding and to communicate your experiences to a healthcare provider to get the support you need.

Maintaining cognitive function during this transition is heavily influenced by diet and exercise. Physical activity is crucial for cognitive health, with numerous studies highlighting its role in boosting memory and executive function. Regular aerobic exercise, such as brisk walking, swimming, or cycling, enhances blood flow to the brain, which is essential for nourishing brain cells and eliminating toxins. Exercise stimulates the production of neurotrophins, proteins that support neuron survival and function, necessary for cognitive health.

Nutrition also significantly impacts brain health. A diet rich in antioxidants, healthy fats, and vitamins supports brain function and mitigates the cognitive effects of menopause. Omega-3 fatty acids — found in fatty fish, flaxseeds, and walnuts —contribute to brain cell integrity. Antioxidant-rich foods such as berries, leafy greens, and nuts combat oxidative stress implicated in cognitive decline. Adequate intake of B vitamins, particularly B12, B6, and folate, is crucial for producing brain chemicals that affect mood and other brain functions. Adapting your diet to include these nutrients enhances clarity and recall.

Incorporating mindfulness and cognitive exercises into your daily routine can help combat brain fog by reducing stress and improving focus and mental clarity. Techniques such as focused breathing, mindful walking, or guided imagery can be easily integrated into your daily schedule, offering moments of mental clarity amid the chaos of menopause. Cognitive exercises— such as puzzles, memory games, or learning new skills—stimulate brain function, helping to keep your mind sharp and responsive.

If brain fog significantly impacts your daily life despite these efforts, it's advisable to consult a healthcare provider. Persistent or worsening cognitive issues may indicate other conditions, such as thyroid dysfunction or vitamin deficiencies, which also affect cognitive function. Navigating through cognitive changes during menopause can be challenging, but clarity can be restored with the right tools and support.

THE TRUTH ABOUT WEIGHT GAIN: METABOLISM AND MENOPAUSE

Weight gain during menopause is a common phenomenon that many women notice, yet it often comes with misconceptions and undue stress. The changes in your body's metabolism due to menopause are real and can be challenging, *but understanding these changes empowers you to manage your weight effectively.* The decrease in estrogen levels that marks menopause impacts your metabolic rate—the rate at which your body uses energy—influences how your body processes fats and carbohydrates. Lower estrogen levels during menopause can slow down metabolism, making it easier to gain weight, especially around the abdomen. This type of fat distribution is linked to higher risks of heart disease and diabetes, making it important to address weight gain for physical appearance and health reasons.

To address metabolic changes, it's important to go beyond calorie counting and incorporate foods that naturally boost metabolism.

Protein-rich foods— such as lean meats, fish, legumes, and dairy— require more energy to digest, increasing the calories burned through digestion. Foods rich in iron and magnesium— spinach, quinoa, and nuts—support healthy thyroid function, which helps regulate metabolism. Minor adjustments such as increasing green tea intake can boost metabolism due to its catechin content.

Hydration is another often overlooked but crucial component. Water is essential for burning calories; even mild dehydration can slow your metabolism. Be sure to drink enough water throughout the day to maintain an optimal metabolic rate.

Exercise is crucial for managing metabolic changes during menopause. Varying your exercise routine and incorporating strength training can help counteract weight gain by increasing your resting metabolic rate. Activities such as weight lifting, yoga, or resistance band exercises can build and maintain muscle. Cardiovascular exercises such as walking, cycling, or swimming are important for burning fat and improving heart health. Tailor your exercise routine to your fitness level and menopause symptoms; for example, low-impact exercises such as swimming or cycling can help if you experience joint pain.

It's essential to embrace body positivity during menopause. Changes to your body's shape and weight are expected during this process. Focus on functional goals such as improving strength, flexibility, or endurance rather than just losing weight. Celebrate what your body *can* do and surround yourself with positive influences. Changing the narrative around menopause and weight can profoundly impact how you experience this phase of your life.

Each strategy you adopt from this chapter on managing your symptoms is a step toward not just coping with menopause but thriving during it. The changes your body undergoes during this time are natural. With the right tools and knowledge, you can adapt to them and thrive.

EMOTIONAL WELL-BEING DURING MENOPAUSE

*N*avigating menopause can be akin to steering through a complex archipelago; each island represents a different aspect of your experience—physical, emotional, and mental. Emotional well-being, though crucial, during menopause is often under-discussed. Understanding and managing your emotional shifts is vital as you traverse this landscape. This chapter explores the deep connection between your hormonal changes and emotional health, offering insights and tools to help you maintain balance and tranquility.

ANXIETY, DEPRESSION, AND MENOPAUSE: BREAKING THE TABOO

The emotional rollercoaster often associated with menopause isn't just a cultural cliché but a reality for many. Hormones like estrogen and progesterone, which are in flux during menopause, don't just regulate your reproductive system; they also influence brain chemicals that control mood. For instance, estrogen impacts neurotransmitters such as serotonin and dopamine, which are essential for maintaining mood stability. As estrogen levels drop, so does the regulation of these neurotransmitters, potentially leading to increased feelings of depression and anxiety. Understanding this biological underpinning is crucial—it's not merely "all in your head" but a profound shift that many women experience during menopause.

Menopausal symptoms—such as sleep disturbances, hot flashes, and physical changes—can contribute to a cycle of stress and anxiety, further exacerbating emotional challenges. The uncertainty about when symptoms will occur and their intensity can itself be a source of anxiety. Recognizing these links helps frame anxiety and depression during menopause, framing them as natural and manageable aspects of the transition rather than stigmatized conditions to be hidden or ignored.

Breaking the Silence

Silence and stigma around menopause can often lead to isolation, making the emotional challenges even harder to bear. Breaking this silence is vital. Open discussions about the emotional aspects of menopause can validate your experiences and provide reassurance that you are not alone. Sharing your feelings with friends, family, or menopause support groups can foster a sense of community and provide emotional relief. These conversations also help spread awareness and understanding about the menopause.

One effective way to initiate dialogue is through community seminars or workshops that focus on the emotional aspects of menopause. These platforms can provide both education and communal support, helping to dismantle the taboos surrounding menopausal emotional health. Such platforms, guided by professionals, provide a safe space to explore your experiences and learn from experts and peers.

Seeking Professional Help

While community support and self-help strategies are valuable, professional help can be crucial, especially for those experiencing severe anxiety or depression. It's important to recognize when it's time to seek help from a healthcare provider or mental health specialist. Symptoms to watch for include persistent sadness, loss of interest in activities you once enjoyed, extreme irritability, or thoughts of self-harm. These signs may indicate the need for professional intervention, including specialized therapies or medications that can help manage these conditions effectively.

Approaching a mental health professional can sometimes feel daunting, but it's an essential step toward taking control of your emotional health. Treatments such as cognitive-behavioral therapy (CBT), counseling, and medication can be tailored to your specific needs, offering relief and new coping strategies. Remember, seeking help is a sign of strength and a proactive step in maintaining your health.

Holistic Approaches

In addition to medical treatments, holistic lifestyle changes can significantly improve your emotional well-being. Regular physical activity, for example, is a powerful antidote to depression and anxiety. Exercise releases endorphins, often called 'feel-good' hormones, which can naturally boost your mood. Activities like yoga, swimming, or brisk walking can be particularly beneficial, offering physical exertion and a mental break from daily stresses.

Nutrition also plays a critical role in emotional health. A balanced diet rich in omega-3 fatty acids, whole grains, and fresh fruits and vegetables can support brain health and improve mood regulation. Reducing the intake of alcohol, caffeine, and sugar—known to exacerbate anxiety and mood swings— can also be beneficial. Integrating healthy approaches into your daily routine can provide a solid foundation for emotional stability during menopause. By addressing both the physical and mental aspects of your health, you create a balanced strategy that supports your overall well-being, allowing you to navigate menopause with vitality and joy.

THE POWER OF MINDFULNESS AND MEDITATION

Finding tranquility during menopause can often feel like searching for calm waters in a stormy sea. However, the ancient mindfulness and meditation practices offer powerful tools to navigate and embrace this phase with a sense of peace and presence. These practices do more than provide temporary relief; they cultivate a deep inner strength that can transform how your experience of menopause. Mindfulness and meditation reduce stress, enhance your cognitive functions, and integrate easily into your daily life, making them essential components of your menopausal wellness toolkit.

Reducing Stress

Stress can exacerbate almost every menopausal symptom, from hot flashes to sleep disturbances. Mindfulness and meditation directly address this by activating your body's relaxation response, a physical state of deep rest that changes your physical and emotional responses to stress. These practices lower the body's stress hormone, cortisol, which is linked to stress and increased abdominal fat, high blood pressure, and impaired cognitive performance. Engaging in mindfulness or meditation can reduce your stress levels, decrease the frequency and severity of menopausal symptoms, and provide a smoother transition.

The beauty of these techniques lies in their simplicity and accessibility. Mindfulness can be practiced anytime, anywhere. It involves paying attention to the present moment without judgment. Whether eating, walking, or simply breathing, mindfulness encourages you to fully immerse yourself in the now, acknowledging and accepting your feelings, thoughts, and bodily sensations. This practice fosters a profound peace that can help relieve the chaotic feelings that often accompany menopause.

Easy Techniques

Incorporating mindfulness and meditation into your daily routine doesn't require special equipment or vast amounts of time. It can be as simple as dedicating a few minutes daily to focus on breathing or practicing mindful awareness during routine activities. For instance, you can practice mindful breathing by concentrating on the sensation of air entering and leaving your body, observing your chest rise and fall, and feeling the air move through your nostrils. This practice can be done for just five minutes in the morning or evening and is a powerful way to center yourself and reduce stress.

Body scan meditation, another accessible technique, involves mentally scanning your body for tension and consciously releasing it. This practice, which starts from the top of your head and moves down to your toes, promotes relaxation by increasing bodily awareness and helping you recognize the early signs of stress or discomfort.

Cognitive Benefits

Mindfulness and meditation can clear 'brain fog' by improving focus, memory, and cognitive flexibility. These practices enhance the brain's ability to process information and adapt to changing situations, skills that are particularly valuable during menopause, when cognitive functions may be under strain.

Research shows that regular meditation leads to changes in brain areas related to attention and memory—such as increased gray matter density in the hippocampus, which plays a key role in learning and memory. These structural changes in the brain enhanced by meditation help maintain and improve cognitive function during and after menopause, helping you retain sharpness and clarity.

Building a Routine

Creating a consistent mindfulness practice tailored to your lifestyle ensures the maximum benefits of these techniques. Start by setting aside a specific time for mindfulness or meditation each day, ideally when you are least likely to be interrupted. Morning, before the day's duties demand your attention, or evening, as a way to unwind before bed, are often well.

Consistency is more important than duration; even a few minutes daily can be beneficial. Create a comfortable space in your home where you can sit quietly without distractions. Include elements that help soothe your senses, such as soft lighting, a comfy cushion, or calming sounds.

Be patient with yourself. Mindfulness is a skill that develops over time, and it's normal to have days when your mind wanders more than it stays present. The goal is not perfection but to develop a deeper understanding and acceptance of your mental patterns, leading to profound insights and emotional balance.

Incorporating mindfulness and meditation into your life reduces stress, enhances cognitive functions, and deepens your relationship with yourself. These practices offer a sanctuary of peace and empower you during the transformative phase of menopause.

JOURNALING THROUGH MENOPAUSE: WRITING AS THERAPY

Of the many tools available for managing the menopausal transition, journaling emerges as a profoundly therapeutic practice. It combines emotional expression, symptom tracking, and personal reflection. Journaling is more than just documenting daily events; it helps you connect with your inner self, explore feelings, and monitor physical health. Writing can unlock emotions and thoughts that are often difficult to articulate verbally, providing a private space for confronting fears, celebrating triumphs, and reflecting on experiences without judgment.

Journaling is a particularly powerful tool for processing emotions. Menopause can introduce a rollercoaster of feelings, from anxiety about physical changes to frustration over fluctuating symptoms. Writing about these emotions helps clarify your feelings and can lead to insights that might not surface otherwise. This process of emotional exploration can be cathartic, relieving stress and offering emotional release. Additionally, journaling about your menopause experience helps you track patterns in your symptoms, offering valuable information that can aid in symptom management. By noting details such as sleep disturbances, mood fluctuations, or the severity of hot flashes, you can identify triggers and understand how various aspects of your lifestyle, diet, or emotional state impact your well-being.

Exploring Journaling Techniques

Different journaling techniques can enhance the benefits of this practice:

> **Gratitude Journaling:** Focuses on acknowledging and appreciating the positive aspects of your life.
> This can be especially beneficial during menopause, a time when challenges can feel overwhelming. Regularly noting things you are grateful for, you cultivate a positive mindset that supports you during tough days.
> **Stream-of-consciousness writing:** Involves free writing without worrying about grammar or coherence. This technique allows you to unload thoughts and feelings that might be cluttering your mind. This liberating writing style encourages you to let go of internal censoring and connect deeply with your emotions.
> **Bullet journaling:** Combines elements of a diary, planner, and to-do list. This method is helpful in tracking menopause symptoms and medications and scheduling self-care activities and appointments.

To begin your journaling journey, consider these prompts:

> "Today, my energy levels were... "
> "A symptom I've noticed lately is... "
> "Today, I felt proud of myself because... "
> "Something that uplifted my mood today was...."

These starters can guide your reflections, making the blank page less daunting and helping you establish a routine that unlocks the therapeutic power of writing.

Consistency is key to fully benefiting from journaling. Set aside a specific time each day for this practice, perhaps in the morning to set a positive tone for the day or in the evening as a way to unwind. Keep your journal in a visible spot to remind you of your commitment to this practice. Treat your journaling time as a non-negotiable appointment with yourself. Over time, journaling can become a cherished ritual that not only helps track your symptoms but also enriches your journey toward self-discovery and emotional resilience.

SELF-IDENTITY AND SELF-ESTEEM: REDISCOVERING YOURSELF

Menopause often ushers in a period of profound change, physically and in how you perceive and feel about yourself. As hormonal shifts reshape, the reflection in the mirror might start to tell a different story than the one you're used to. This evolving narrative can stir a range of emotions—from confusion to liberation—affecting your sense of identity and self-esteem. It's natural to ask, "Who am I now?" as you notice the changes in your body and perhaps your thoughts and feelings. This period of adjustment also presents a valuable opportunity for rediscovery and redefining who you are and how you see yourself.

Knowledge is power, and understanding the biological and psychological aspects of menopause can demystify the process. Navigating these changes often starts with a clear understanding of menopause itself. Learning about menopause isn't just about recognizing the symptoms but also about understanding the naturalness of this transition, which every woman experiences uniquely. This can transform your perspective, enabling you to see this phase as a new chapter of life with opportunities for growth and rediscovery. Armed with the right information, you can make more informed decisions about your health and lifestyle and significantly boost your confidence.

Engaging in new or revisited activities can significantly enhance your self-esteem during menopause. Activities that challenge you physically or intellectually can provide a sense of accomplishment and purpose, whether it's taking up a new sport, learning a new language, or exploring a creative hobby like painting or writing. These endeavors reinforce your capabilities, reminding you of your strengths and talents, which the focus on menopausal symptoms might have overshadowed. These activities offer a constructive distraction from the discomforts of menopause, providing relief and a sense of normalcy and continuity in your life.

The role of body positivity during this time cannot be overstated. Menopause can change how your body looks and feels, and these changes can sometimes challenge your body image and self-esteem. Embracing these changes with kindness and acceptance is crucial. Shifting your focus from how your body looks to what it can do and celebrating it for its strength and resilience. Practicing body positivity might involve simple affirmations reinforcing self-love or participating in social groups celebrating body diversity and empowerment. Remember, the changes you experience during menopause are natural. Maintaining a positive attitude and practicing self-compassion can foster a healthier body image and strengthen your self-esteem.

Building a supportive environment helps immensely in cultivating a positive self-image during menopause. Surrounding yourself with people who understand and support your experience can make a significant difference. This support network can provide both emotional comfort and practical advice and insights, which can be invaluable. Engaging in open conversations about menopause with friends, family, or support groups not only aids in your own adaptation process but also helps normalize menopause as a natural stage in life, reducing stigma and promoting a more inclusive understanding of this transition.

As you adjust to menopause, remember this is a time for rediscovery. You are not losing your identity but evolving it. With each change, you can learn more about yourself, redefine your self-image, and develop a renewed sense of who you are. Embrace this time with curiosity and compassion, and allow yourself to explore and enjoy becoming more authentically you.

RECLAIMING YOUR JOY AND FINDING HAPPINESS

While managing the physical and emotional changes that menopause brings, it's vital to remember the importance of joy and happiness in your life. These elements are not just extras; they are essential to your well-being. During menopause, you might find that the sources of joy you once relied on no longer resonate with you in the same way. This doesn't mean that joy has become elusive; it might simply mean it's time to rediscover what brings you happiness now. This part of your life offers a unique opportunity to reconnect with old passions or discover new interests that ignite joy and excitement.

Identifying what brings you joy might seem daunting, especially if you've been focused on navigating symptoms or changes. Start by reflecting on moments in your day when you feel at peace or find yourself smiling effortlessly. These moments can provide clues to what brings you joy. For some, it might be spending time in nature; for others, it could be creative expression like painting or writing; or for you, it might be spending quality time with loved ones. Once you identify these sources, incorporate them into your daily life. It could be as simple as scheduling a weekly walk in the park, joining a local art class, or setting regular dates with friends or family.

Hobbies and social activities significantly enhance your quality of life during menopause. Staying active isn't just about physical health; it's about keeping your mind and spirit engaged. Finding pursuits that challenge you or learning new skills can be enjoyable and give you a sense of achievement and purpose. Whether it's gardening, photography, cooking, or volunteering, these activities can substantially boost your mood and self-esteem. They also keep your mind engaged and allow you to interact with others who share your interests, which can be incredibly fulfilling.

The concept of gratitude has gained much attention in recent years for its positive impact on mental health and overall well-being. Cultivating a practice of gratitude during menopause can significantly shift your perspective, helping you focus on the positive aspects of your life. This practice involves regularly acknowledging things you are grateful for, no matter how small. Try keeping a gratitude journal, listing daily entries of things you appreciated that day. You could make it a habit to think of three things you're grateful for each morning or share them with a family member each evening. Over time, this practice can shift your focus from what you feel you have lost to appreciating what you have, enhancing your overall sense of well-being.

Joy in connection with others is particularly valuable during menopause when you might feel misunderstood or isolated due to the changes you're experiencing. Building and maintaining solid relationships with friends and family can provide emotional support and joy. These connections offer comfort, understanding, and validation of your experiences. They can be a source of fun and laughter, which are wonderful antidotes to stress and anxiety. Don't hesitate to reach out to old friends or make new connections, perhaps by joining clubs or groups that align with your interests. Remember, sharing your experiences with others who understand or are going through similar changes can make your menopausal phase much more manageable and enjoyable.

Embracing joy and happiness during menopause involves actively seeking and engaging in activities that bring pleasure, cultivating an attitude of gratitude, and nurturing connections with others. Integrating these practices into your life enhances your emotional well-being and transforms your menopausal experience into a more positive and fulfilling phase. This proactive approach to finding joy and happiness enriches your life and empowers you to navigate menopause with optimism and resilience.

BUILDING A SUPPORTIVE COMMUNITY: YOU'RE NOT ALONE

A supportive community during menopause is a crucial element that can profoundly influence how you navigate this transition. The importance of a robust support network cannot be overstated—it provides emotional solace, practical advice, and a sense of belonging that can reduce feelings of isolation or confusion that sometimes accompany menopause. As you find your way through the varied experiences of menopause, having a tribe, a group of people who understand and support you, can be your anchor and guide.

Finding your tribe might seem intimidating, especially if you feel that those around you might not understand what you're going through. However, numerous ways exist to connect communities that resonate with your needs. Online platforms, for instance, offer a wealth of resources and networks. Websites and forums dedicated to menopausal support not only provide information but also connect you with women worldwide who are at various stages of this transition. These virtual spaces allow for sharing experiences and advice, ensuring you have access to a community no matter your location. Social media groups are another vibrant resource where daily interactions can help you feel connected and supported, offering instantaneous communication with peers who can provide empathy and insights in real time.

Local support groups and health clinics sometimes host menopause workshops or meetings, providing a space to meet others face-to-face. These gatherings can be particularly enriching because they allow for real-time interaction and the formation of friendships with those who might be in the same geographic area. If such groups are not available in your area, consider starting one. Libraries, community centers, and even cafes can be great places to host such meetings. Engaging with your community not only helps you but also creates a space for others who might be seeking the same support.

The role of family in this phase of your life is also paramount. Menopause doesn't have to be a solitary journey—having your family understand and support you can significantly ease the transition. This might require open conversations with your partner, children, or other close family members about menopause and how it affects you. Educating them about your needs and the changes you are experiencing can foster empathy and help them provide the support you need, whether it's understanding your mood swings, helping around the house, or simply being there to listen when you need to talk. Family can be your first line of support, playing a critical role in how positively you navigate menopause.

Giving back to your community can also be a powerful way to foster a supportive network. Volunteering your time, knowledge, or resources to support other women experiencing menopause can be incredibly rewarding. It not only helps them but can also give you a sense of purpose and belonging. Organizing informative talks, sharing your experiences, or even providing a listening ear can make a huge difference in someone else's life. Giving back creates a positive feedback loop within your community, enhancing your sense of well-being while helping others through their transitions.

Building these networks, remember that the support you seek can often start with you extending your hand first. By reaching out, sharing your story, and being there for others, you lay the foundations of a community that uplifts and sustains its members through the challenges of menopause.

From understanding the deep connection between your hormonal changes and emotional health to engaging in therapies like mindfulness and journaling and building a supportive community, each step is designed to ensure that you maintain not just your physical health but also your emotional and mental well-being. These strategies can hold you steady through the ebbs and flows of menopause.

∼

RELATIONSHIPS AND INTIMACY

As the tides of menopause rise and fall, so too can the dynamics of your relationships and intimacy. This chapter explores how menopause can recalibrate your connections, particularly with your partner. You might find yourself on a path where open communication becomes your compass, guiding you through uncharted waters of change with your partner. Explore how deepening your dialogue can illuminate your menopause journey and the paths you share with your partner.

COMMUNICATION IS KEY: TALKING ABOUT MENOPAUSE WITH YOUR PARTNER

Initiating a conversation about menopause with your partner may feel daunting. Starting this dialogue is essential in nurturing understanding and empathy within your relationship. Begin by choosing a comfortable setting where you feel safe and relaxed—perhaps during a quiet evening at home or on a leisurely walk. It's helpful to start the conversation broadly, perhaps by sharing how you've been feeling lately, before gradually introducing specific topics related to menopause. Acknowledge that while this might be a new subject for both of you, it's important. Encourage a two-way dialogue from the start. Choose a time when neither of you are rushed or stressed, ensuring the conversation isn't overshadowed by external pressures but is instead a dedicated space for open, honest communication.

Educating Your Partner

As you ease into these discussions, it becomes evident that sharing knowledge about menopause can be incredibly enlightening for your partner. Many people are unaware of the breadth of symptoms and their impacts. Take the opportunity to explain the physiological changes, such as hot flashes or sleep disturbances, and the emotional fluctuations you might be experiencing. This education can be eye-opening, shifting from mere awareness to a deeper understanding of your daily realities. Utilize resources such as books, reputable websites, or even consultations with healthcare providers you can attend together. This shared learning journey can strengthen your bond as it transforms menopause from a personal challenge into a shared chapter of your lives.

Expressing Needs and Desires

Expressing your needs and desires during menopause is crucial. This phase can alter your emotional landscape significantly, requiring different forms of support from your partner. Be clear about what support is most meaningful to you, whether it's physical comfort during a hot flash or a patient listener when you're feeling down. Equally important is inquiring about your partner's needs. They may also be experiencing confusion, fear, or concern as they watch you navigate menopause, and acknowledging their feelings validates that this is a shared experience. This mutual exchange fosters a deeper emotional connection, reinforcing that your relationship can adapt and thrive through these changes.

Navigating Changes Together

Approaching menopause as a team can turn potential hurdles into opportunities for growth. Discuss strategies for managing changes together, such as adjusting your lifestyle to accommodate new sleep patterns or finding new ways to connect emotionally and physically. Flexibility and patience are your allies; what works one month might need adjustment the next. Celebrate small victories and recognize that while menopause is a significant life event for you, it's also one you are navigating together. This approach deepens your bond and cultivates a shared resilience that can weather this and other challenges.

By fostering a supportive and empathetic dialogue with your partner, you lay a foundation of mutual respect and understanding that enhances your connection, ensuring that you both feel valued and supported as you adapt to the changes together.

REVIVING INTIMACY: BEYOND VAGINAL DRYNESS AND LIBIDO CHANGES

Many women experience changes in their sexual health during menopause, which can be both confusing and distressing. One of the most common physical changes is vaginal dryness, a direct result of decreased estrogen levels. This decrease affects the vaginal tissues, making them less elastic and more susceptible to irritation. Fluctuations in libido are also common, influenced by both physiological and psychological factors during menopause. It's essential to approach these changes with knowledge and compassion, recognizing them as natural and manageable aspects of your evolving body.

To address the discomfort of vaginal dryness, a variety of lubricants and moisturizers are available that can significantly enhance comfort during intimate moments. Water-based lubricants are popular for their compatibility with natural body tissues and latex condoms, providing moisture without causing irritation. Silicone-based lubricants offer longer-lasting lubrication and can be a good option for women who find water-based products insufficient. For those who prefer a more natural approach, coconut oil is an effective alternative that many find effective, though it should not be used with latex condoms as it may cause them to break down. Regular use of vaginal moisturizers, which are designed to mimic natural vaginal secretions, can help maintain moisture and elasticity for both intimate and daily comfort.

Exploring new avenues of intimacy can also rejuvenate your connection with your partner during menopause. Intimacy extends beyond physical interactions; it encompasses emotional and intellectual connections that can be equally fulfilling. Discussing books, sharing music, or engaging in creative activities together can strengthen your bond and provide new shared experiences that enhance closeness. Physical intimacy may evolve to include more cuddling, massage, or simply holding hands—gestures that maintain a physical connection without the pressure of sexual performance. This broader understanding of intimacy embraces the changes menopause brings, allowing you and your partner to explore new dimensions of closeness that adapt to your current needs and desires.

Sometimes, the changes in intimacy during menopause may benefit from professional guidance. Sex therapy or couples counseling can help navigate the complex emotions and adjustments that accompany menopausal changes in intimacy. A qualified therapist can offer strategies to improve communication about sexual needs and concerns, helping you and your partner navigate this sensitive area with understanding and care. Therapy can also provide a space to explore emotional blocks or anxieties that might be affecting your sexual relationship, offering tools to rebuild intimacy in ways that are respectful and satisfying for both partners.

Maneuvering the physical changes of menopause concerning intimacy requires patience, open communication, and sometimes a willingness to redefine what intimacy means for you and your partner. By addressing these changes proactively, whether through lubricants, exploring new forms of closeness, or seeking professional advice, you can maintain a fulfilling, intimate relationship that adapts to the natural progression of life's phases. This approach enhances your relationship and supports your overall well-being as you move through menopause with confidence and grace.

SOLO AND THRIVING: NAVIGATING MENOPAUSE WITHOUT A PARTNER

Like many of life's significant phases, menopause presents unique challenges and opportunities. For those going through this transition without a partner, the experience might seem daunting. However, it also opens up a profound space for personal growth and self-discovery. Embracing menopause solo can be a powerful journey toward deepening your self-care practices and reinforcing your independence. Focusing on your well-being and learning to meet your needs can enhance your quality of life and empower you to live fully and satisfyingly.

Self-care is not just an occasional indulgence—it's an essential practice, especially during menopause. For those navigating menopause without a partner, self-care becomes even more important. It's about creating a lifestyle that supports your physical, emotional, and mental health. Establishing a routine that incorporates nutritious meals, regular physical activity, and sufficient sleep are fundamental aspects that can help mitigate menopausal symptoms such as fatigue, mood swings, and hot flashes. Beyond the physical, self-care also means setting aside time for activities that nourish your soul and bring you joy, whether reading, gardening, or artistic pursuits. It also involves allowing yourself to rest and retreat when needed, listening to your body's cues without guilt. Mindfulness or meditation can further enhance your self-care regimen, allowing you to connect with your inner self and easily navigate emotional highs and lows.

Expanding your social network is another enriching aspect of thriving solo during menopause. Building and maintaining strong social connections are vital—they can provide emotional support, enhance your sense of belonging, and keep loneliness at bay. Explore new groups or clubs in your community that align with your interests. Whether it's a book club, a hiking group, or a crafting circle, these are spaces where you can meet new people who share similar passions. Volunteering is another rewarding way to expand your social circle while giving back to the community.

Volunteering can connect you with people from diverse backgrounds and age groups, enriching your social experience and providing a broader perspective on life. Engaging in social activities helps build friendships and boosts your social confidence, which can be incredibly empowering during a time of change like menopause.

Personal growth is perhaps the silver lining of navigating menopause solo. It's a perfect time to reevaluate your life's goals and what truly matters to you. Perhaps there are personal or professional aspirations you put on hold; menopause can be the catalyst you need to pursue these dreams with renewed vigor. Consider furthering your education by taking a course or attending workshops that pique your interest. Exploring new hobbies or reviving old ones can also be tremendously fulfilling. These activities enrich your life with new skills and knowledge and bolster your independence and self-esteem. They remind you that personal growth is a lifelong process, and menopause is another stage where you can flourish and expand your horizons.

Embracing sexuality with confidence is equally crucial, especially when you are experiencing menopause without a partner. Understanding your sexual needs during this time can be both liberating and enjoyable. Self-exploration can be valuable, allowing you to understand your body's changes and discover what brings you pleasure. This might include exploring self-pleasure through new techniques or toys, enhancing your sexual experience, and promoting a healthy sexual relationship with yourself. Remember that sexuality does not diminish with age; instead, it evolves and can be a profoundly affirming part of your menopause experience.

Facing menopause without a partner offers a unique opportunity to reinvest in yourself across many levels—from deepening your self-care practices and expanding your social life to pursuing personal growth and embracing your evolving sexuality. Each aspect contributes to a holistic approach to menopause, which honors where you are in life and celebrates where you are heading. By focusing on nurturing yourself and your relationships, you can turn this period of transition into one of empowerment and personal renewal, filled with opportunities for growth and joy.

MENOPAUSE AND FRIENDSHIP: DEEPENING BONDS

Friendships play a crucial role in your life, and during menopause, their importance can become even more pronounced. As you navigate the fluctuations of menopause, friends can act as anchors, providing comfort, laughter, and a listening ear when most needed. These relationships often grow during times of change, as friends offer support, understanding, and companionship vital for emotional health. Nurturing these bonds during menopause can lead to deeper, more meaningful friendships.

Empathy stands at the heart of deepening these friendships. It's the bridge that connects your experience to someone else's, allowing for a deeper understanding and stronger connections. During menopause, when your emotions and physical experiences can feel particularly intense, having friends who empathize with what you are going through can be incredibly comforting. Empathy in friendships fosters a safe space where you can express vulnerabilities without fear of judgment. This mutual understanding can transform casual friendships into deeper bonds, creating a supportive network that celebrates successes and provides comfort during challenges.

Shared experiences are another cornerstone of strengthening friendships during menopause. These experiences, whether they relate directly to menopause or broader aspects of life, can deepen bonds and provide mutual support. Consider joining or forming a menopause support group where you can share and learn from others at a similar stage in life. These groups can be invaluable for connecting with others who understand exactly what you are going through. Alternatively, simple shared activities such as regular walks, yoga classes, or craft sessions can also be bonding opportunities. These activities not only allow you to spend quality time together but also promote a sense of camaraderie and mutual support, reinforcing your connections.

Incorporating wellness and relaxation into your outings with friends can enhance your bonds while promoting a healthy lifestyle. Activities such as spa days, meditation retreats, or wellness workshops provide relaxation and enjoyment and create shared memories that can bring you closer together. These experiences are fun and investments in your collective well-being, providing a break from the daily routine and an opportunity to recharge together. Planning these activities can be collaborative, allowing everyone involved to contribute ideas and preferences, further strengthening the group dynamic.

Expanding your circle of friends to include new acquaintances who are also navigating menopause can bring fresh perspectives and additional support. Meeting new people at a similar life stage can be incredibly refreshing and help you feel less isolated in your experiences. Look for local clubs, online forums, or community classes to meet a diverse group of women. Welcoming new friends into your life expands your support network and enriches your menopausal experience with varied insights and stories. These new relationships can invigorate your social life and provide fresh energy, reminding you that menopause is a universal experience.

Reflect on the invaluable role that friendships play in your life, especially during menopause. The bonds you nurture now can offer comfort, joy, and a more profound sense of community. Remember, the empathy you share, the experiences you enjoy together, and the new friendships you forge during this time are not just sources of support; they are powerful affirmations of the shared human experience.

Navigating menopause involves adapting your relationships, intimacy, and personal growth. Open communication with your partner, exploring new dimensions of intimacy, and embracing self-care are essential. Whether you're navigating this transition solo or with a partner, focusing on nurturing relationships and expanding your social network can turn menopause into an opportunity for empowerment and personal renewal. By addressing these aspects proactively, you can enhance your well-being and embrace this transformative phase with confidence and grace.

DIET AND NUTRITION

The foods you choose can be your allies during the ebbs and flows of menopause, helping to temper the tides of hormonal fluctuations and symptom flare-ups. This chapter explores nutritional strategies to support your body through transition, focusing on how specific foods can alleviate symptoms and enhance your overall well-being. By adjusting your dietary habits, you're nourishing your body and supporting your journey through menopause.

FOODS THAT FIGHT HOT FLASHES AND SUPPORT HORMONAL BALANCE

During menopause, lower estrogen levels can bring a host of symptoms, hot flashes being among the most common and disruptive. Fortunately, nature offers its bounty in the form of phytoestrogens —plant-derived compounds that mimic the effects of estrogen. Foods rich in phytoestrogens, such as soy and flaxseeds, can supplement the body's loss of estrogen.

Soybeans—and soy products, like tofu and tempeh—contain isoflavones, a type of phytoestrogen that has been shown to have a mild estrogenic effect, helping to moderate temperature regulation and reduce hot flashes. Flaxseeds boast lignans (a different kind of phytoestrogen) and omega-3 fatty acids, contributing to their anti-inflammatory properties. Incorporating these foods into your diet can be as simple as blending ground flaxseeds into your morning smoothie or adding tofu into your meals several times a week. The key is consistency, as the benefits of phytoestrogens are most pronounced when included as part of a regular dietary pattern.

Calcium and Vitamin D: Pillars of Bone Health

Calcium and vitamin D are vital in maintaining bone health, particularly during menopause, when the risk of osteoporosis increases. As estrogen levels drop, bone resorption accelerates, leading to a decrease in bone density. Calcium is a critical building block of bone tissue, and vitamin D is essential for calcium absorption and bone growth.

Dairy products are well-known sources of calcium, but if you're dairy-free, there are plenty of alternatives. Leafy greens like kale, broccoli, and fortified plant milks or juices are excellent sources. Vitamin D, often called 'sunshine vitamin,' is synthesized in the skin through sunlight exposure. Still, factors like the winter season or high latitudes might limit your ability to produce enough. Foods like fatty fish (such as salmon and mackerel), egg yolks, and fortified foods can help fill the gap. Consider discussing vitamin D supplementation with your healthcare provider to ensure adequate levels.

Balanced Fats for Hormonal Health

The role of fats in hormonal health is often misunderstood. Certain fats, particularly omega-3 fatty acids, are crucial in managing menopause symptoms and overall hormonal balance. Omega-3s, found in fish like salmon and sardines and seeds such as chia and hemp—are known for their anti-inflammatory properties. They can help combat the inflammatory responses associated with menopause, such as joint pain or skin changes. These fats are also crucial for brain health, which can be beneficial as you navigate mood swings or memory issues. Including a moderate amount of healthy fats in your diet can also aid in satiety, helping to manage weight by keeping you fuller for longer.

Magnesium-Rich Foods: Supporting Sleep and Mood

Magnesium, a mineral praised for its versatility in health support, deserves a spotlight in your menopausal diet. It plays a vital role in over 300 enzymatic reactions in the body, including sleep and mood—two areas often affected during menopause. Magnesium helps activate the parasympathetic nervous system, which calms and relaxes the body. This action can be particularly beneficial if you suffer from sleep disturbances. Magnesium also interacts with neurotransmitters that are responsible for calming the brain and promoting relaxation, aiding in mood regulation. Turn to green leafy vegetables (spinach and Swiss chard), legumes, nuts, seeds, and whole grains to boost your magnesium intake. These foods are rich in magnesium and provide other nutrients that support overall health, making them excellent additions to a menopause-friendly diet.

THE SUGAR CONNECTION: BLOOD SUGAR, MOOD SWINGS, AND MENOPAUSE

Navigating menopause often means managing hormonal fluctuations and the intricate balance of your blood sugar levels. It's not unusual to experience mood swings and sudden energy crashes during this time, symptoms that can be exacerbated by blood sugar instability. Understanding the connection between your diet and controlling your blood sugar is crucial for easing these symptoms. When your blood sugar levels fluctuate widely, it can trigger hormonal changes that may worsen menopause-related symptoms, particularly mood swings. By stabilizing your blood sugar through dietary choices, you can achieve a more balanced emotional and physical state.

The key to stabilizing blood sugar is to focus on the quality and types of carbohydrates in your diet. High glycemic index (GI) foods, such as white bread, sugary drinks, and pastries, can cause rapid spikes in blood sugar, followed by equally rapid declines, which can send your energy levels and mood on a roller coaster ride. Opt for low-GI alternatives—foods that cause a steady, more controlled increase in blood sugar—to maintain more stable blood sugar levels throughout the day. Foods such as whole grains, legumes, most fruits, and non-starchy vegetables are excellent low-GI choices that contribute to blood sugar stability and provide vital nutrients and fiber, enhancing overall health.

Incorporating these low-GI foods into your daily meals doesn't have to overhaul your diet drastically. Start with simple swaps: choose brown rice or quinoa instead of white rice; opt for whole-grain bread over white bread; snack on fruits and nuts instead of cookies or chips. These changes, while small, can significantly impact how your body processes sugar, helping to keep your mood and energy levels more consistent. Integrating these foods into your diet also supports your cardiovascular health—a crucial consideration during menopause, when the risk of heart issues can increase.

Avoiding Sugar Traps

Becoming adept at reading food labels is invaluable. Processed and packaged foods often contain hidden sugars, which can disrupt your efforts to control blood sugar control. It is essential to learn to identify these sugars under their many names—such as sucrose, high-fructose corn syrup, and dextrose. This enables you to make informed choices about the products you consume, steering clear of those that might contribute to blood sugar spikes.

Opting for natural sweeteners can also be a strategic choice in managing your sugar intake. Options like stevia, which comes from the leaves of the Stevia plant, or monk fruit sweetener offer sweetness without the blood sugar impact of regular sugar. These alternatives can be beneficial if you want to reduce your sugar intake without sacrificing sweetness, whether in your coffee, tea, or home-baked goods. However, use these sweeteners sparingly to reduce your overall reliance on sweet tastes, helping to reduce cravings over time.

The Role of Fiber

Fiber plays a multifaceted role in your diet because it regulates digestion and supports steady blood sugar levels. High-fiber foods, such as legumes, whole grains, fruits, and vegetables, slow down sugar absorption in your bloodstream, preventing the spikes and drops that can affect your mood and energy. A fiber-rich diet can also aid in weight management—a common concern during menopause—by increasing feelings of fullness and reducing overall calorie intake.

To enhance your fiber intake, incorporate a variety of fiber-rich foods into each meal. Start your day with oatmeal topped with berries, enjoy a lunch with a quinoa salad with mixed vegetables, and end with a dinner featuring a hearty lentil soup or a stir-fry loaded with fibrous veggies. Snacking on nuts, seeds, or raw vegetables between meals can also boost your fiber intake, keeping hunger and blood sugar levels in check.

By understanding and managing the sugar connection through dietary choices that stabilize blood sugar, focusing on low-GI foods, smartly navigating food labels, and prioritizing fiber, you can significantly ease the mood swings and energy crashes often associated with menopause. These dietary strategies enhance your immediate well-being and contribute to long-term health benefits that extend beyond menopause. Remember that each meal is an opportunity to support your body through this significant phase of life, crafting a dietary pattern that nourishes and sustains you daily.

GUT HEALTH AND HORMONES: THE UNSEEN LINK

Understanding the intricate relationship between your gut health and hormonal balance during menopause is often overlooked. The gut microbiome plays a pivotal role in how your body adapts and responds to the hormonal shifts that characterize this stage of life. The microbiome—a complex community of bacteria residing in your digestive system—influences everything from your metabolism to your immune system and even your mood. During menopause, its role in estrogen metabolism becomes particularly significant. Estrogen is processed in your reproductive organs and metabolized in your gut. Healthy gut bacteria can convert estrogen into forms that your body can use effectively, helping to maintain a balance that relieves some of the more challenging symptoms of menopause.

An imbalance in these gut bacteria, often referred to as dysbiosis, can lead to inefficient estrogen metabolism and exacerbate menopausal symptoms such as hot flashes, weight gain, and mood swings. Incorporating a variety of probiotics and prebiotics into your diet can foster a thriving gut environment that supports your hormonal health throughout menopause. Probiotics—found in fermented foods like yogurt, kefir, sauerkraut, and kimchi—introduce beneficial bacteria to your gut. These foods aid in digestion and help in producing and regulating critical hormones and neurotransmitters. Prebiotics—found in fibrous foods such as bananas, onions, garlic, and asparagus—help nourish your gut bacteria, ensuring they can thrive and perform their necessary functions.

The anti-inflammatory properties of a well-maintained gut can be a boon during menopause. Inflammation is a natural immune response, but when chronic, it can lead to numerous health issues, including exacerbated menopausal symptoms. An anti-inflammatory diet focuses on foods that support gut health and reduce inflammation. Omega-3 fatty acids, for instance, are potent anti-inflammatory agents. While often highlighted for their benefits to heart and brain health, their impact on gut health and inflammation is equally significant. Foods rich in omega-3s—flaxseeds, chia seeds, and fatty fish such as salmon—can help reduce the inflammatory responses in your body, aiding in symptom relief. Antioxidants play a crucial role in combating inflammation. Colorful fruits and vegetables, rich in antioxidants, can help neutralize free radicals in your body, reducing oxidative stress and inflammation.

Making these dietary adjustments to improve gut health need not be overwhelming. Start small; introduce one new probiotic or prebiotic food into your diet each week—experiment with incorporating anti-inflammatory foods into your meals in simple, enjoyable ways. Add slices of avocado to your morning toast, include a handful of berries in your yogurt, or swap out your usual cooking oil for extra virgin olive oil. These small changes can become part of your daily routine, significantly improving your gut health and menopause journey. By nurturing your gut microbiome through thoughtful dietary choices, you're supporting your digestive health and creating a hormonal environment that can help smooth menopause transitions.

SUPPLEMENTS AND MENOPAUSE: SEPARATING FACT FROM FICTION

In the landscape of menopause management, dietary supplements often appear as beacons of hope, promising relief from the pervasive symptoms. While some supplements have garnered attention for their potential benefits, it's crucial to approach them with a well-informed perspective, understanding their possible advantages, limitations, and risks. Supplements like black cohosh and red clover have become synonymous with natural menopause relief. Black cohosh has been widely studied for its effectiveness in reducing hot flashes and improving mood swings. Derived from a plant native to North America, it is thought to work by influencing serotonin receptors and mimicking some effects of estrogen in the body. While some studies suggest benefits, others have found it no more effective than a placebo, highlighting the variability in individual responses to herbal supplements.

Red clover, another popular choice, contains isoflavones, plant-based chemicals that produce estrogen-like effects in the body. It is often used to ease symptoms such as hot flashes and night sweats. The research on red clover is mixed, with some studies indicating modest benefits while others suggest minimal impact. This discrepancy can be attributed to differences in the study designs, the dosages used, and the specific menopausal symptoms addressed. The effectiveness of these supplements can vary widely among individuals, influenced by factors such as age, the severity of symptoms, and individual health conditions. While these supplements can be part of a broader strategy to manage menopause symptoms, they should not be relied upon as the sole treatment method.

Safety and efficacy are paramount when considering any supplement. The allure of 'natural' treatments can sometimes overshadow the need for rigorous scrutiny regarding their safety. Both black cohosh and red clover are generally considered safe for short-term use but are not without side effects. Black cohosh has been associated with liver issues in rare cases, while red clover can increase the risk of bleeding, particularly in women taking blood-thinning medications. Given these potential risks, the importance of consulting healthcare providers before starting any new supplement regimen cannot be overstated. This step ensures you consider any underlying health conditions and medications that might interact negatively with the supplement.

Discussing your plans with a healthcare provider can provide additional guidance tailored to your specific health needs and menopausal symptoms. Healthcare providers can offer insights into the latest research and recommend supplements with a track record of safety and efficacy. They can also help you establish a clear, personalized plan for supplement use, including optimal dosages and durations tailored to your health profile and menopausal symptoms.

Navigating the world of supplements also requires awareness of potential interactions with other medications. Supplements can sometimes interfere with the way your body processes medications, either diminishing the medication's effectiveness or exacerbating its side effects. For example, St. John's Wort, commonly used for mood management during menopause, can interact with a variety of medications, including antidepressants, birth control pills, and blood thinners, potentially leading to serious health consequences. Supplements like ginkgo biloba, which some women take for memory and concentration, can increase the risk of bleeding if taken with certain anti-inflammatory drugs or anticoagulants.

This complex interplay of interactions underscores the necessity of a cautious, informed approach when integrating supplements into your menopause management plan. It's not enough to consider the potential benefits of a supplement; understanding how it interacts with other aspects of your health care is equally crucial. By discussing your options with healthcare professionals and thoroughly researching each supplement, you can make informed decisions that enhance your well-being without compromising your safety. Supplements can serve as a valuable complement to other lifestyle and dietary strategies, forming a holistic approach to managing menopause that respects the complexity of your body's needs during this transformative phase.

HYDRATION: THE OVERLOOKED HERO OF MENOPAUSE MANAGEMENT

Amid the complex strategies to manage menopause symptoms, hydration stands out for its simplicity and impact. Water is essential, yet its importance often gets overshadowed by more specific dietary adjustments. During menopause, your body's need for water increases as changes in hormone levels can enhance fluid retention and dehydration risks. These changes can manifest in various ways, from dry, itchy skin to more frequent urinary tract infections and noticeable vaginal dryness. Each of these conditions speaks to the body's cry for more hydration—a call that, when answered, can alleviate some of the most persistent menopausal discomforts.

Managing hydration begins with setting daily water intake goals. The general recommendation is to drink at least eight 8-ounce glasses of water daily, which equates to about 2 liters or half a gallon. However, this is just a starting point; factors such as weight, activity level, and overall health can influence your needs. A practical approach to ensuring you meet your hydration needs is to observe the color of your urine; it should be light yellow. Darker urine can indicate dehydration. To facilitate this, consider starting your day with a large glass of water and keeping a reusable water bottle with you throughout the day, making it easier to sip regularly. You might also set reminders on your phone or computer, prompting you to hydrate periodically and turning water consumption into a habit that seamlessly fits into your daily routine.

Incorporating hydrating foods into your diet can significantly contribute to your fluid intake. Cucumbers, melons, and berries are rich in water and packed with vitamins, minerals, and antioxidants that support overall health. Cucumbers, for instance, are about 95% water and can be easily added to salads or eaten as a refreshing snack. Melons, including watermelon and cantaloupe, are similarly hydrating and provide a sweet, nourishing treat. While slightly lower in water content, berries are both hydrating and high in fiber, which can support bowel health—a bonus during menopause when digestive processes may slow down. Including these foods in your daily diet enhances your hydration and adds a burst of flavor and nutrients, making your meals more enjoyable and more supportive of your body's needs during menopause.

However, it's just as crucial to be aware of and moderate your intake of dehydrators—substances that can increase fluid loss. Caffeine and alcohol are prime examples, both of which can have a diuretic effect, leading to increased urine production and potential dehydration. While you don't have to eliminate these entirely, moderation is key. Pay attention to how your body responds to these substances. Reducing your caffeine intake, particularly in the form of coffee or soda, and limiting alcoholic beverages, particularly those high in sugar, can help maintain your hydration levels. Opting for herbal teas or diluting juices with water can provide healthier alternatives that keep you hydrated without contributing to fluid loss. You can maintain optimal hydration by setting realistic daily water intake goals, incorporating hydrating foods into your diet, and moderating dehydrators. As simple as it may seem, water becomes a cornerstone of your dietary strategy during menopause, supporting your body's needs in a natural, accessible way.

From understanding the benefits of phytoestrogens to stabilizing your blood sugar levels, enhancing gut health, and navigating the world of supplements, each piece of nutritional advice in this chapter aims to help you with the knowledge to make informed choices. Additionally, staying hydrated and mindful of your gut health will further contribute to your well-being. With the proper nutrition and support, you can empower yourself to navigate this transition confidently and healthily.

EXERCISE AND PHYSICAL HEALTH

*E*xercise is not just a routine; it's a celebration of what your body can achieve and a powerful tool for easing the transitions that menopause brings. It involves moving in ways that feel good and align with your body's changing needs. This chapter will guide you in creating an exercise regimen tailored to your lifestyle and menopausal symptoms, helping you maintain agility, strength, and happiness.

EXERCISE THAT WORKS: TAILORING YOUR ROUTINE TO YOUR SYMPTOMS

The relationship between exercise and menopause is symbiotic; each enhances the other. Customizing your exercise routine to address specific menopausal symptoms can transform your approach to physical activity. For instance, yoga is celebrated for its physical benefit and ability to reduce stress and promote relaxation, making it ideal for managing stress-related symptoms of menopause. The gentle stretches and mindful breathing integral to yoga help soothe the nervous system, lower cortisol levels, and foster a sense of calm and control amid the hormonal upheaval.

On the other end of the spectrum, weight-bearing exercises are essential in maintaining bone health, a major concern during menopause due to the increased risk of osteoporosis. Activities such as walking, jogging, dancing, and lightweight training help strengthen muscles and bones by working against gravity. Integrating these exercises into your routine can help mitigate bone density loss, a subtle yet significant effect of menopause.

Starting small is key to integrating exercise into your life without feeling overwhelmed. Begin with what feels manageable—perhaps a 10-minute daily walk or a few yoga poses each morning—and gradually increase the duration and intensity as your comfort and fitness levels improve. This gradual approach helps build a sustainable exercise habit without the risk of injury or burnout, which can be higher during menopause due to physical changes and increased sensitivity to stress.

Variety in your exercise regimen is crucial to covering the spectrum of health benefits needed during menopause. Incorporating a mix of cardiovascular, strength, and flexibility exercises ensures a holistic approach to your physical health. Cardiovascular exercises, such as swimming or cycling, boost heart health and improve endurance, while flexibility exercises, such as stretching or Pilates, improve mobility and reduce the risk of injury. This variety not only addresses multiple health concerns but keeps your routine engaging, which is essential for long-term motivation.

Speaking of motivation, staying inspired to keep moving can sometimes be a challenge, especially on days when menopausal symptoms are more pronounced. Setting realistic goals, tracking progress, and celebrating small victories can be very motivating. Whether it's increasing the duration of your walk, mastering a new yoga pose, or simply feeling more energetic, acknowledging these achievements can propel you forward. Finding an exercise buddy or joining a class can further boost your commitment, making exercise an enjoyable part of your routine rather than a chore.

By incorporating these strategies, physical activity becomes a powerful, personalized tool for managing menopause. Selecting and varying your activities ensures that your routine is comprehensive, enjoyable, and specifically tailored to alleviate your menopausal symptoms, transforming exercise into a pathway for enhancing your quality of life during menopause.

STRENGTHENING YOUR CORE: THE KEY TO PELVIC HEALTH

The muscles around your trunk and pelvis—your core—are fundamental to your overall health, especially during menopause. A strong core supports virtually every movement and is crucial for maintaining balance and stability. Equally important is the health of your pelvic floor, a group of muscles that supports the pelvic organs and is responsible for urinary control. During menopause, hormonal changes can weaken these muscles, potentially leading to incontinence—a common but often unspoken issue for many women during menopause. Strengthening your core and pelvic floor can significantly improve your quality of life.

Understanding the connection between a strong core and improved pelvic health is essential. The core muscles, including the transversus abdominis, obliques, and rectus abdominis, work in harmony with the pelvic floor muscles. When these muscles are strong, they help maintain proper posture and alignment, vital for the functioning of the pelvic organs. A robust core and pelvic floor provide the support needed to prevent accidental urine leakage during activities like coughing, sneezing, or lifting. Moreover, strengthening these muscles can enhance your sexual health, contributing to sexual function and satisfaction.

To strengthen these critical areas, incorporating specific core exercises into your routine is essential. Pelvic tilts and bridges are two effective exercises that target your core and engage and strengthen the pelvic floor muscles. A pelvic tilt involves lying on your back with your knees bent and feet flat on the floor. Gently arch your lower back and roll your hips toward your head. This movement engages the lower abdominal muscles and the pelvic floor. The bridge pose involves lying in the same starting position but lifting your hips toward the ceiling, creating a straight line from your shoulders to your knees. This exercise strengthens the lower back and abdominal muscles while providing a good workout for the pelvic floor. Regularly practicing these exercises can significantly enhance muscle tone and control, offering a strong defense against the pressures that menopause places on pelvic health.

Incorporating these exercises into your daily activities can further enhance muscle strength. For instance, consciously engaging your core and pelvic muscles while sitting at a desk or walking can train these muscles to stay active throughout the day, enhancing muscle memory and strength. Incorporating breathing techniques focusing on diaphragmatic breathing can further strengthen the core and pelvic floor. When you breathe deeply, your diaphragm moves, creating a gentle pressure that naturally engages these muscles and provides an ongoing low-intensity workout.

If you face challenges with pelvic floor health, consult a physical therapist specializing in pelvic floor rehabilitation. These professionals can create a tailored program that targets your core and pelvic floor muscles and guide you on proper techniques to maximize your exercises safely.

Strengthening your core and pelvic floor during menopause is not just about physical health; it's an investment in your autonomy and confidence during this transformative phase. By focusing on targeted exercises and seeking professional guidance when needed, you can ensure that menopause is a phase marked by strength rather than vulnerability.

YOGA AND MENOPAUSE: A NATURAL SYMPTOM SOOTHER

Yoga, a practice steeped in rich tradition, offers more than just physical benefits; it provides a sanctuary for those navigating the complexities of menopause. This ancient practice tones the body and soothes the soul, making it an ideal choice for managing various menopausal symptoms. Imagine engaging in a practice that aligns your physical movements with your breath, creating a balance that can alleviate discomforts such as hot flashes, insomnia, and mood swings. Its gentle, fluid movements help cool down internal heat, which is particularly beneficial for managing hot flashes. Many yoga poses also promote better sleep patterns, combating the insomnia that is often associated with menopause.

The power of yoga in reducing stress and enhancing emotional equilibrium is significant. Through specific breathing techniques known as Pranayama, yoga teaches you to harness the power of your breath to manage stress and mood swings. One such technique, the Ujjayi breath, involves breathing deeply through the nose with a slight constriction at the back of the throat, enhancing relaxation and reducing cortisol levels, which are often elevated during menopause. Incorporating these breathing exercises into your daily routine can help you maintain a calm, centered state of mind, significantly improving your mental well-being.

Restorative yoga poses are especially beneficial for menopausal women. These poses promote relaxation and stress relief, using props such as cushions, blankets, and blocks to support the body in a comfortable position. For example, Child's Pose (Balasana) is a gentle pose that can help to calm the mind and relieve tension in the body, making it ideal for when you feel overwhelmed or exhausted. Legs-Up-The-Wall (Viparita Karani) involves lying on the floor with your legs extended vertically against a wall. This pose improves circulation and helps to reduce night sweats while calming the nervous system and promoting better sleep.

Incorporating daily yoga into your routine can be a gentle yet powerful way to address the physical and emotional challenges of menopause. If you are new to yoga, finding a class that suits your needs is important. Beginning classes focus on gentle poses and provide personalized guidance to ensure a safe place. Some studios and online platforms offer classes specifically designed for menopausal women, emphasizing poses and breathing techniques that are effective for symptom relief.

Online resources provide tutorials and routines for those who prefer to practice at home. Websites and apps like YogaGlo or Gaia offer a variety of classes you can follow in the comfort of your home.

Starting with just a few minutes of yoga daily can significantly affect how you feel. You can gradually extend your practice as you become more comfortable with the poses. Remember consistency and listening to your body is key; yoga is about finding balance and peace, not perfection.

Yoga offers a natural approach to managing menopause, soothing both body and mind. Its benefits extend beyond physical health, nurturing emotional and spiritual well-being, and helping you navigate menopause with grace and strength.

OUTDOOR ACTIVITIES: FRESH AIR FOR FRESH PERSPECTIVES

Embracing the outdoors during menopause is like turning a fresh page every day; each experience breathes new life into your routine and brings myriad benefits to both your mind and body. Nature offers a sanctuary where the simple act of stepping outside can make you feel better. Whether a leisurely walk in the park, an invigorating hike, or a peaceful hour spent gardening, connecting with the natural world can bolster your physical health and emotional resilience during menopause.

One immediate benefit of outdoor activities is the exposure to vitamin D, often called the 'sunshine vitamin.' As estrogen levels decline during menopause, your body needs increased vitamin D to maintain bone density and boost your mood. Regular sunlight exposure can naturally increase your vitamin D levels, combating the risk of osteoporosis. Vitamin D plays a role in modulating mood, warding off depression, and strengthening your bones, making outdoor activities a double boon for your health.

Spending time in nature also reduces stress. Natural settings have a unique ability to enhance calm and relaxation. The serene sights and sounds—the rustling leaves, the chirping birds, and the gentle breezes—contribute to lowering stress hormones such as cortisol. Activities such as hiking through a forest or walking along a beach can be particularly meditative, helping to align your movements and breathing for a tranquil state of mind. This connection with nature can shift your focus away from daily stresses and menopausal discomforts, providing a refreshing reset for your mind.

The options are plentiful for those looking to incorporate more outdoor activities into their lifestyle. Hiking combines physical exercise with the sensory pleasures of the outdoors. It engages your cardiovascular system, strengthens your muscles, and, depending on the terrain, can be a challenge that boosts your endurance. Not all hikes need to be strenuous; many trails are designed with varying levels of difficulty, and even a gentle hike can offer substantial health benefits. Cycling is another excellent option, providing a cardiovascular workout that is easier on the joints than running. Cycling through a park or along a dedicated bike trail can be a joyful activity that elevates your heart rate and spirits.

Gardening is a rewarding outdoor activity that combines physical activity with the calming effects of being in nature. It involves bending, stretching, digging, and pulling, enhancing flexibility and strength. Gardening also offers the satisfaction of nurturing growth, which can be incredibly rewarding and therapeutic. Watching something you planted grow and thrive provides a profound sense of accomplishment and a connection to the cycle of life—especially comforting during menopause.

Incorporating outdoor activities into your daily life doesn't require major planning. It can be as simple as walking to your local store instead of driving, spending a few minutes of your lunch break in a nearby park, or dedicating part of your weekend to a nature trail or garden. The key is to make these activities a regular part of your life, allowing the cumulative benefits of fresh air, sunlight exposure, and nature's calming effects to enhance your menopause journey. As you embrace the outdoors, you'll find that nature serves as a backdrop for exercise and a refreshing resource that supports your health and well-being.

THE IMPORTANCE OF BONE HEALTH: PREVENTING OSTEOPOROSIS

Understanding the dynamics of bone health during menopause is crucial, as the risk of osteoporosis increases at this stage. As estrogen levels drop, bones may lose calcium and other minerals more rapidly, leading to decreased density and increased fragility over time, which raises the risk of fractures. Early prevention and understanding of bone density loss are essential for managing health during menopause.

Maintaining bone density involves a combination of diet, exercise, and regular health assessments. A diet rich in calcium and vitamin D is fundamental for bone health. Dairy products such as milk, cheese, and yogurt are rich in calcium, which is essential for bone strength. For those who are lactose intolerant or vegan, fortified plant-based milk, green leafy vegetables, and almonds are excellent alternatives. Vitamin D, critical for calcium absorption, can be obtained from sunlight. However, with aging, the skin's ability to convert sunlight into vitamin D decreases, which may necessitate supplementation as advised by a healthcare provider.

Incorporating weight-bearing exercises into your routine is also vital. Activities like walking, jogging, dancing, or lifting weights require the body to work against gravity, stimulating the growth of bone cells. Strength training helps maintain muscle mass and bone density. Aim for at least 30 minutes on most days of the week, gradually increasing intensity to avoid injury. These exercises also improve balance and coordination, which can help prevent falls—a common risk factor for bone fractures among menopausal women.

Regular screening for bone density is another pivotal aspect of maintaining bone health. Bone density tests can assess bone health and determine the rate of bone loss. Regular bone density screenings are essential for assessing bone health and monitoring bone loss rates. By keeping track of your bone health, you and your healthcare provider can make informed decisions about interventions, such as lifestyle changes or medications. Women are encouraged to start these screenings around the onset of menopause, especially if they have risk factors such as a family history of osteoporosis, a petite body frame, or a history of smoking.

Navigating the complexities of bone health during menopause doesn't have to be daunting. By integrating calcium-rich foods and vitamin D into your diet, embracing weight-bearing exercises, and following a regular screening schedule, you can take proactive steps to safeguard your bones, prevent osteoporosis, and lead a vibrant, active life beyond menopause.

CARDIOVASCULAR CARE: WHY HEART HEALTH MATTERS MORE NOW

As you navigate through menopause, understanding your cardiovascular health becomes increasingly crucial. It's a lesser-known fact that women's risk of heart disease tends to rise after menopause. This increase is due to the declining estrogen levels. It plays a critical role in maintaining the elasticity of arteries, helping to keep blood pressure in check. As estrogen levels drop, your arteries may become stiffer, potentially leading to higher blood pressure and heart strain. Additionally, changes in blood lipid profiles—such as increased LDL (bad) cholesterol and decreased HDL (good) cholesterol—can further elevate this risk. These shifts highlight the importance of focusing on heart health during and after menopause to maintain vitality and well-being.

Incorporating heart-healthy exercises into your routine is one of the most effective strategies for supporting cardiovascular health during menopause. Activities such as brisk walking, cycling, and swimming are particularly beneficial. These exercises rhythmically engage large muscle groups, improving the efficiency of your heart and lungs. Over time, regular cardiovascular exercise can help lower your heart rate and blood pressure, reduce the risk of heart disease and stroke, and enhance your overall heart health. The simplicity and accessibility of these activities —whether it's a brisk walk in your neighborhood, a cycle through a local park, or a swim at your community pool—make them easy to incorporate into your daily life.

A heart-healthy diet is essential in cardiovascular care during menopause. Focus on whole grains, lean proteins, and plenty of fruits and vegetables while minimizing the intake of saturated fats and processed foods. Whole grains such as oatmeal, quinoa, and whole wheat bread are rich in fiber, which helps lower cholesterol levels. Lean proteins, including fish, poultry, and legumes, provide essential nutrients without high saturated fats in some red meats. Various fruits and vegetables ensure a rich intake of antioxidants and other heart-protective nutrients. Limiting the intake of high-fat, high-salt, and high-sugar foods can help prevent spikes in blood sugar and blood pressure, which is particularly important when your cardiovascular system is already facing the challenges of menopause.

Managing stress is another critical aspect of cardiovascular care. Chronic stress can lead to adverse health effects, including an increased heart rate and blood pressure, which put a strain on the cardiovascular system. Techniques such as meditation and deep breathing exercises can be powerful tools for reducing stress. Meditation helps you focus and calm your thoughts, lowering stress hormones. Deep breathing exercises such as diaphragmatic breathing encourage full oxygen exchange and help lower or stabilize blood pressure.

By engaging in regular cardiovascular exercise, adhering to a heart-healthy diet, and managing stress, you equip yourself with the tools to support your heart health through menopause and beyond. This proactive approach mitigates the increased risk of heart disease associated with menopause while enhancing your overall quality of life, helping you to remain active, energetic, and joyful in your postmenopausal years. Remember that each step toward cardiovascular care is a step toward a healthier, more vibrant you.

FINDING YOUR FIT: ADAPTING YOUR EXERCISE ROUTINE TO YOUR CHANGING BODY

As your body navigates menopause, adapting your exercise routine to accommodate physical changes is essential. During menopause, your body undergoes significant transformations that can influence everything from joint health to muscle elasticity. It's not uncommon for women to experience increased joint sensitivity or decreased bone density during this time, making high-impact activities like running less appealing or even uncomfortable. Shifting to lower-impact exercises such as swimming, cycling, or using an elliptical machine can help maintain cardiovascular health while minimizing joint stress.

Menopause can bring about shifts in weight distribution and muscle tone, which might impact your balance and strength. Activities that focus on building core strength, balance, and flexibility become increasingly important. For example, Pilates can be an excellent choice—it focuses on the core, which in turn helps improve balance and overall stability. Resistance training with bands or light weights can help maintain muscle mass, which naturally declines with age. Incorporating these forms of exercise can help you feel stronger and more in control of your body despite the changes it is going through.

Maintaining an active lifestyle during menopause can sometimes be challenging due to a lack of motivation, time constraints, or physical discomfort. Overcoming these barriers begins with setting achievable, clear goals and integrating exercise into your daily routine in a way that feels rewarding rather than burdensome. For instance, if time is limited, you might start with exercises you can do during daily activities like calf raises while washing dishes or squats during television commercials. Having a workout buddy can provide a significant boost for those days when motivation is lacking. It also introduces an element of accountability, which can be incredibly motivating.

Exploring new activities and sports that resonate with your current life stage can also renew your enthusiasm for physical activity. This may be an opportunity to discover interests that align with your evolving physical capabilities. For example, you might take up dancing, which provides a cardiovascular workout, enhances coordination, and lifts the spirit. With their gentle movements and focus on breath control, Tai chi or qigong can offer both physical and mental health benefits. These low-impact activities can be adapted to various fitness levels and mobility issues that may arise during menopause.

Setting realistic goals is essential to maintain motivation and ensure that the benefits of exercise are enjoyable. Goals should be specific, measurable, achievable, relevant, and time-bound (SMART). Instead of setting vague goals like 'get fit,' aim for specific targets such as 'attend three yoga classes per week' or 'walk for 30 minutes every day.' These precise goals are easier to manage and track, leading to a greater sense of accomplishment and encouraging you to stick with your routine. Celebrating these small victories can boost your confidence and inspire you to keep moving forward, helping you adapt to your changing body and lifestyle.

Navigating the physical changes during menopause requires a flexible approach to exercise that accommodates your body's needs while supporting vitality and wellness. By adapting your exercise routines, exploring new activities, and setting realistic goals, you cater to your body's needs and enhance your overall quality of life during this transformative phase. Remember the importance of listening to your body and responding with kindness. The strategies discussed in this chapter—from adjusting your exercise types to setting achievable goals—can help you maintain an active and fulfilling lifestyle through menopause and beyond.

UNDERSTANDING HORMONE REPLACEMENT THERAPY (HRT)

Hormone Replacement Therapy (HRT) often emerges in discussions about menopause as a potential source of relief, yet it remains enveloped in controversy and misunderstanding. Imagine finding a key that could unlock comfort and well-being during menopause, but know that the key must be used with caution and awareness. That is what HRT represents for many women navigating menopause. This chapter aims to clarify the complexities of HRT, offering a clear understanding of what it is, how it works, and how it can be integrated into your menopause management plan.

DEMYSTIFYING HRT: THE BASICS

Hormone Replacement Therapy (HRT) is a treatment used to replenish the estrogen levels that naturally decline during menopause. Its primary goal is to alleviate the symptoms caused by reduced estrogen, which include hot flashes, night sweats, vaginal dryness, and mood swings. By restoring these hormones, HRT can significantly ease these symptoms and enhance the quality of life for many women.

Forms of HRT

HRT is not a one-size-fits-all solution; it comes in various forms and dosages, allowing for personalized treatment plans. Common forms include pills, patches, gels, and creams. Each form has its delivery method and rate of absorption, which can influence both effectiveness and side effects. For example, estrogen pills are taken orally and pass through the liver before entering the bloodstream. In contrast, patches and gels provide a direct dose through the skin, resulting in a steadier absorption rate and potentially fewer side effects. The chosen form of HRT depends on individual factors, such as personal preference, specific symptoms, and overall health profile.

HRT and Symptom Relief

The efficacy of HRT in symptom relief is well-documented. Estrogen pills can reduce hot flashes and night sweats by up to 75 percent and can also improve sleep, mood, and joint pain. Vaginal estrogen—available as creams, tablets, or rings—is particularly effective for treating vaginal dryness, discomfort during intercourse, and some urinary symptoms. While HRT can significantly improve daily functioning and overall well-being, understanding both its benefits and potential risks is crucial for making an informed decision that aligns with your health goals.

Starting HRT

Beginning HRT should involve a thorough discussion with your healthcare provider, who can evaluate your medical history, discuss your symptoms, and discuss the potential risks and benefits. This conversation should cover HRT's different forms and dosages to find the most suitable option for you. Typically, the lowest effective dose is often recommended to minimize potential risks. Regular follow-ups are essential to monitor the therapy's effectiveness and make any necessary adjustments. Starting HRT is a significant decision in managing your health during menopause, and understanding all aspects of this therapy is crucial.

WEIGHING THE RISKS AND BENEFITS OF HRT

When considering Hormone Replacement Therapy (HRT), it's crucial to have a balanced view of the potential risks and the benefits it offers. This dual perspective ensures informed decision-making regarding your unique health needs and life circumstances.

Starting with the risks, it's well-documented that HRT, especially certain types and dosages, can be associated with an increased risk of breast cancer, heart disease, and stroke. These risks vary depending on whether estrogen is administered alone or with a progestin, your current age, the age at which menopause began, and the duration of the hormone therapy. For instance, using combined hormone therapy for more than five years has been shown to elevate the risk of breast cancer slightly. It's also noted that this risk returns to normal once hormone therapy has been discontinued for several years. Similarly, the risk of heart disease and stroke can increase, particularly if HRT is started more than ten years after menopause onset or after the age of 60. This underscores the importance of timing in the initiation of HRT.

Risks: HRT, particularly certain types and dosages, can be associated with an increased risk of breast cancer, heart disease, and stroke. Risks vary depending on age, age at menopause onset, the duration of therapy, and whether estrogen is used alone or in combination with progestin. Using combined hormone therapy for over five years can slightly elevate the risk of breast cancer, though this risk returns to normal after discontinuation for several years. Heart disease and stroke risks can also increase, especially if HRT is started more than ten years after menopause onset or after age 60. Timing is key when considering HRT.

Benefits: The primary benefit of HRT is alleviating severe symptoms such as hot flashes and night sweats, particularly when therapy is started early in menopause. Estrogen therapy after menopause can also improve bone density, lowering the risk of osteoporosis and fractures.

The decision to use HRT is personal and should be based on a detailed assessment of your risks, which varies significantly among women. Factors such as age, your family history of diseases like breast cancer or heart disease, and your personal medical history should be considered. For instance, if you are at higher risk for blood clots, a transdermal patch may be a safer option than pills because it delivers hormones directly into the bloodstream, bypassing the liver and potentially reducing the risk of clotting.

Ongoing monitoring and adjustments are integral parts of managing HRT effectively. Once HRT is initiated, regular follow-ups with your healthcare provider are crucial. These check-ins provide an opportunity to adjust the dose or method of delivery based on your symptoms and any side effects you might be experiencing.

Additionally, regular screenings for breast cancer, heart disease, and other relevant conditions are recommended to manage potential risks proactively. These screenings are essential to your overall health monitoring while on HRT. They ensure that any adverse effects are identified and addressed promptly.

The decision to start HRT involves careful consideration of multiple factors, including your personal health history, familial risks, and the severity of your menopausal symptoms.-This decision-making process should be revisited regularly as your health needs and circumstances evolve. Engaging openly with your healthcare provider, armed with knowledge about the risks and benefits, prepares you to make an informed choice. Remember, the ultimate goal is to enhance your quality of life during menopause and beyond. Deciding on HRT is a medical consideration and a potential stepping stone to health and vitality.

HRT AND CANCER RISK: WHAT YOU NEED TO KNOW

Navigating the complexities of Hormone Replacement Therapy (HRT) involves a critical understanding of cancer risks, an aspect that often raises concerns. Recent studies and continuous research provide insights into how HRT can impact the risk of developing certain types of cancer, notably breast and ovarian cancers. This understanding is vital for making informed health decisions regarding HRT usage during menopause.

The correlation between HRT and breast cancer has been one of the most extensively studied. Research indicates that the risk of breast cancer can vary significantly based on the type of HRT, the duration of use, and individual health history. For instance, estrogen-only HRT generally poses less risk than combined HRT, which includes both estrogen and progesterone. Studies have shown the risk associated with HRT tends to decrease once the therapy has been discontinued for several years, pointing to the importance of personalized treatment durations and monitoring.

Ovarian cancer risk, while less commonly discussed, is also influenced by HRT. The risk increase is generally considered to be smaller compared to breast cancer but is still significant enough to warrant careful consideration. The duration of HRT plays a key role with regard to ovarian cancer, with longer durations generally associated with higher risks.

The decision to undergo HRT should be based on a thorough evaluation of your personal and family medical history. If your family history includes instances of breast or ovarian cancer, this information is crucial in determining your baseline risk levels. Genetic factors, like mutations in the BRCA1 or BRCA2 genes, which significantly increase the risk of breast and ovarian cancers, are also critical in this assessment. A comprehensive evaluation, including genetic testing, can provide a clearer picture of how HRT might influence your cancer risk profile.

For those concerned about the cancer risks associated with HRT, it's important to discuss alternatives without the use of hormones. While detailed options will be discussed later, it's worth noting that non-hormonal medications, lifestyle modifications, and certain herbal supplements can significantly manage symptoms. For instance, certain antidepressants have been effective in reducing hot flashes, while changes in diet and exercise have been shown to improve overall health and help manage weight.

Understanding the intricate relationship between HRT and cancer risks is more than just recognizing the potential dangers. It involves understanding how personalized medical care, informed by the latest research, can help navigate these risks. This empowers you to make decisions that align with your health priorities and lifestyle while ensuring your approach is as safe and effective as possible.

PERSONAL STORIES OF HRT: VARIED EXPERIENCES

The diverse experiences of countless women shape the narrative of Hormone Replacement Therapy (HRT). The personal stories shared in this section are real-life experiences illuminating the outcomes of HRT. These stories are vital, as they echo the scientific data and bring to life the personal and sometimes complex decisions women face regarding HRT.

Maria – Taming Hot Flashes and Night Sweats

Maria, a 52-year-old schoolteacher, started HRT as she entered menopause. Maria's initial symptoms included severe hot flashes and night sweats that not only disrupted her sleep but also began to affect her performance at work. After a detailed consultation with her doctor, weighing the benefits and potential risks, Maria decided to start on a low-dose estrogen patch. The change wasn't immediate, but within a few months, Maria noticed a significant reduction in her symptoms. Her sleep improved dramatically, and she felt more like her old self at work. For Maria, HRT was transformative, enhancing her quality of life when she needed it most. Her story is a testament to the potential positive impact of HRT when it is carefully considered and tailored to an individual's symptoms and health profile.

Jenna – Mood Swings and Side Effects

Jenna, a 48-year-old graphic designer, opted for HRT due to persistent mood swings that affected her relationships. She chose a combined hormonal pill, a decision influenced by her desire to stabilize her hormonal fluctuations quickly. Initially, she felt relief from the emotional rollercoasters, but over time, she experienced side effects such as headaches and minor weight gain. This prompted several discussions with her healthcare provider, leading to adjustments in her treatment. Jenna's story emphasizes a critical aspect of HRT—the need for ongoing monitoring and flexibility in managing HRT treatments, acknowledging that adjustments may be necessary as the body responds differently over time.

Sarah – Impact of Family Health History

Sarah, a 50-year-old freelance writer, wrestled with the decision to start HRT because her mother had battled breast cancer. She engaged in multiple discussions with her healthcare providers and underwent genetic screenings and risk assessments to understand her risks thoroughly. She opted for nonsystemic vaginal estrogen therapy to minimize hormone exposure to her body while addressing her severe urogenital symptoms. Sarah's proactive approach underscores the importance of tailoring HRT to individual symptoms and health history.

Each narrative reflects a different facet of the HRT experience, from life-changing benefits to the necessity for adjustments and the deep considerations required when family health history and risks are involved. These stories serve as a potent reminder of the individual nature of health care. What works for one may not work for another, and the best decisions are always made when armed with comprehensive information and supported by professional guidance. As you consider your path through menopause and whether HRT might be a part of that journey, let these stories remind you of the power of informed choice and the importance of closely monitoring and adjusting any treatment plan.

ALTERNATIVES TO HRT: WHAT ELSE YOU CAN TRY

For those seeking alternatives to HRT, various options stand out as effective strategies. Many women, whether due to personal health histories, preferences, or specific concerns about HRT, seek out these options.

Nonhormonal Medications: Selective Serotonin Reuptake Inhibitors (SSRIs) have been recognized for their effectiveness in mitigating some of the psychological symptoms associated with menopause, such as mood swings and depressive states. SSRIs increase serotonin levels in the brain, a neurotransmitter that helps boost mood and reduce feelings of sadness or anxiety. Originally developed to treat depression, SSRIs have been found to significantly alleviate emotional fluctuations during menopause, offering a pharmacological option for women who are unable or unwilling to use hormone therapy. Always discuss the potential side effects and interactions with other medications with your healthcare provider to determine their appropriateness for you.

Lifestyle Modifications: A balanced diet of fruits, vegetables, whole grains, and lean proteins supports overall health during menopause. Regular physical activity—including cardiovascular, strength training, and flexibility exercises—helps manage weight, improve mood, and enhance quality of life. Stress management techniques such as yoga, meditation, and deep-breathing exercises can also alleviate symptoms such as hot flashes and improve sleep quality. These lifestyle changes not only help in managing the physiological and psychological aspects of menopause but also contribute to long-term health and well-being.

Natural Supplements: Phytoestrogens, found in plants like soy and flaxseeds, mimic the effects of estrogen in the body and can help balance hormone levels. Herbs such as black cohosh, known for its potential to ease menopausal symptoms, and St. John's wort, which may help with mood swings and depression. Always consult a healthcare provider before using supplements, as they are not strictly regulated and can interact with prescribed medications.

Combining these various approaches—nonhormonal medications, lifestyle modifications, and natural supplements—into a cohesive management plan offers a flexible and personalized approach to dealing with menopause without HRT. While these alternatives to HRT provide viable options for many women, it is essential to consult with healthcare professionals before starting any new treatment.

Remember that each woman's menopause experience is unique, and what works for one may not work for another. Embracing menopause with the informed choices discussed in this chapter, supported by professional advice and personal research, can lead to effective symptom management and improved quality of life. This holistic approach addresses immediate discomforts and long-term health, paving the way for sustained vitality in later years.

∼

NATURAL & ALTERNATIVE REMEDIES AND COMPLEMENTARY THERAPIES

As you navigate the transformative waves of menopause, you may find solace in nature's offerings. Whether it's the calming presence of herbal tea or the therapeutic effects of carefully selected supplements, natural remedies can provide gentle support through the ebbs and flows of hormonal changes. This chapter explores how herbal allies can gracefully support you through menopause. We'll delve into the world of herbal helpers, from the forested hills where black cohosh grows to the fields of red clover and the ancient gardens of Dong Quai. These herbs have been harnessed for centuries to ease women's transitions through different life stages. Here, we gather their secrets, backed by scientific evidence, to help you incorporate these natural remedies into your daily regimen.

HERBAL HELPERS: A GUIDE TO SUPPLEMENTS AND TEAS

Herbal medicine offers a variety of options, but knowing which herbs are effective for alleviating menopausal symptoms can guide you toward making informed choices. Black cohosh, an herb native to North America, has traditionally been used by Native Americans for women's health issues. Today, it is widely recognized for its potential to alleviate hot flashes and mood swings associated with menopause. Red clover, rich in isoflavones, mimics estrogen in the body, providing a natural way to balance balance hormones gently. Dong Quai, often called 'female ginseng,' is a cornerstone of traditional Chinese medicine, valued for managing menstrual discomfort and menopausal symptoms.

Each of these herbs offers unique benefits, and incorporating them into your routine can provide natural relief during menopause. However, the effectiveness of these herbs can vary based on factors such as herb quality, the preparation method, and your body chemistry. Consulting a healthcare provider knowledgeable in herbal medicine can help you choose the right herbs for your specific needs.

Safety and Dosage

While herbal supplements have many benefits, safety and correct dosing must be fundamental. Natural does not always mean safe; herbal potency can vary dramatically depending on the source and preparation. For instance, the dosage of black cohosh should be carefully monitored, as excessive intake has been linked to liver issues. Start with the lowest possible dose and adjust gradually under the guidance of a healthcare professional. Also, herbs such as Dong Quai can interfere with blood thinners and other medications, making discussing potential interactions with your healthcare provider essential.

Scientific Evidence

Scientific research supports the traditional use of herbs, although results can be inconsistent. Clinical trials on black cohosh have produced mixed results regarding its effectiveness in reducing hot flashes, suggesting that it may work better for some women than others. Similarly, studies on red clover indicate that it can help reduce the frequency and severity of hot flashes. Reviewing the latest research and consulting with a healthcare provider can help you understand the current findings related to the efficacy of these herbs in managing menopausal symptoms.

Teas for Symptom Management

Adding herbal remedies into your daily routine can be as delightful as sipping a warm cup of tea. Herbal teas offer a comforting, soothing way to benefit from herbs. Chamomile tea, known for its calming properties, can help manage mood swings and sleep disturbances. Green tea, rich in antioxidants, may lower the risk of osteoporosis and heart disease. Regularly drinking these teas can be an effective, simple way to introduce beneficial herbs into your system, promoting relaxation and overall well-being.

ACUPUNCTURE AND MENOPAUSE: PINPOINTING RELIEF

Acupuncture, a practice rooted in Traditional Chinese Medicine (TCM), provides a unique approach to managing menopausal symptoms. Dating back thousands of years, acupuncture is based on the concept of Qi (pronounced "chee"), the vital life force or energy that flows through the body. TCM views health as a harmonious balance of this energy, and illness or discomfort—such as those experienced during menopause—are seen as imbalances or blockages in Qi flow. The process involves inserting thin, sterile needles at specific points along the body's energy pathways, or meridians. Acupuncture aims to restore balance, encourage healing, and support the body's natural ability to regulate its processes, including those disrupted during menopause.

The practice of acupuncture is grounded in the holistic view of the body, which does not isolate symptoms but treats the whole system. For example, in TCM, the liver is seen as the organ responsible for the smooth flow of blood throughout the body. Similarly, the kidney, associated with aging and vitality in TCM, often focuses on treating symptoms like night sweats and hot flashes. Acupuncture's nuanced, organ-centered approach offers a personalized and integrative treatment option during menopause.

Exploring the science behind acupuncture reveals its complexity and profound potential. Studies suggest that acupuncture points are conductors of electromagnetic signals. Stimulating these points enables the release of endorphins, the body's natural painkillers, and affects the brain's ability to regulate serotonin levels, which influences mood and sleep. Additionally, acupuncture may influence the hypothalamus and pituitary gland, stabilizing hormone levels during menopause. Acupuncture's potential to naturally modify hormone fluctuations is what draws many to consider it a viable option for menopause management.

The evidence supporting the effectiveness of acupuncture in relieving menopausal symptoms continues to grow. One study published in the journal *Menopause* found that women who received acupuncture experienced a notable decrease in the frequency and severity of hot flashes. Another study pointed to improvements in sleep patterns among menopausal women undergoing acupuncture, attributing these changes to the treatment's ability to influence melatonin production.

Finding a qualified and experienced acupuncturist trained in TCM is essential for safely integrating this therapy into your menopause management plan. Some countries and regions have regulatory boards that oversee acupuncturists' certification and practice standards, ensuring they meet specific educational and professional criteria. When choosing an acupuncturist, don't hesitate to ask about their training, approach, and previous patient outcomes. A good practitioner will also offer guidance on complementary lifestyle changes and self-care practices.

THE ROLE OF AROMATHERAPY AND ESSENTIAL OILS

Aromatherapy, with its rich palette of scents derived from nature's essence, offers a soothing and holistic approach to managing the diverse and often challenging symptoms of menopause. This ancient practice, based on essential oils extracted from flowers, herbs, and trees, taps into the profound connection between scent and well-being. Aromatherapy works at a deep cellular level by engaging our olfactory system to provide relief and comfort. Essential oils possess properties that can influence both the body and mind to address the hormonal imbalances and emotional rollercoasters experienced during menopause.

Among the many types of essential oils, clary sage and lavender stand out for their specific benefits in alleviating menopausal symptoms. Clary sage is known for its ability to balance hormones, and its calming aroma is particularly effective in soothing stress and promoting a sense of well-being. Studies have shown that inhaling clary sage can significantly decrease cortisol levels, the stress hormone that often spikes during menopause. Lavender, celebrated for its relaxing properties and soothing scent, has been shown to lower heart rate and blood pressure, promoting relaxation and better sleep.

Essential oils can be utilized in a variety of ways. Diffusers-disperse the oil's molecules into the air. Adding a few drops of lavender or clary sage to a diffuser before bedtime can transform your bedroom into a sanctuary conducive to restful sleep. Topical application of oils-can be beneficial for targeted relief. Mixing clary sage with a carrier oil such as jojoba or almond and massaging it into the abdomen can alleviate menstrual-like cramps. Similarly, applying lavender oil to the temples or wrists can help ease tension headaches and soothe nerves.

Another vital aspect of aromatherapy is creating a calm environment. Beyond merely smelling pleasant, aromatherapy creates an atmosphere that nurtures and heals. Imagine drawing a warm bath after a long day and adding a blend of bergamot, known for its uplifting properties, and ylang-ylang, which promotes relaxation. Incorporating this holistic approach into your daily rituals can elevate these moments into relaxation and reflection opportunities.

However, as with any potent remedy, proceed with caution. Essential oils are highly concentrated and must never be applied directly to the skin without diluting in carrier oil. This prevents potential skin irritations and enhances the oil's efficacy as the carrier oil helps to absorb the essential oils into the skin better. Some oils can have contraindications with medications or existing health conditions. For instance, rosemary oil, while beneficial for enhancing memory and concentration, should be used cautiously by those with hypertension or epilepsy. Consulting with a professional, especially when you are just beginning to explore the world of essential oils, is advisable to tailor your aromatherapy experience to your specific health needs.

As you continue to explore and experience the fragrant world of essential oils, remember that this journey toward alleviating menopausal symptoms is about finding what works and enjoying the process, one soothing scent at a time. Whether through a diffuser, a bath, or a personal inhaler, these fragrant oils can transform your menopausal experience into one of tranquility and balance.

MASSAGE THERAPY: MORE THAN JUST RELAXATION

The soothing power of touch through massage therapy offers significant benefits during menopause. It addresses physical and emotional symptoms such as anxiety, joint pains, and bouts of depression. The rhythmic pressure and strokes applied during a massage can significantly alleviate these discomforts, facilitating a more profound sense of well-being and physical ease.

A primary benefit of massage therapy is its effectiveness in reducing anxiety and enhancing mood. This is achieved by stimulating serotonin and dopamine, neurotransmitters that play critical roles in stabilizing mood. These chemicals are naturally released during a massage session, helping to create feelings of calm and contentment while simultaneously reducing cortisol levels. This stress hormone is often elevated during menopause. This hormonal balance not only helps soothe anxiety but can also mitigate other symptoms of menopause, such as irritability and mood swings. Additionally, massage therapy can be a boon for physical ailments such as joint pain, a common complaint as estrogen levels, which help reduce inflammation and decline during menopause. During a massage, manual manipulation of muscles and joints enhances blood flow, relieves muscle tension, and promotes pain relief by releasing endorphins, the body's natural painkillers.

Exploring the different types of massage therapy can help you choose the one that works best for you. Swedish massage induces relaxation and improves circulation by using long, flowing strokes combined with kneading and tapping techniques on the outer layers of muscles, making it perfect for relieving muscle tension and stress. Deep tissue massage may be more appropriate if deep-seated tension or chronic pain points are among your concerns. This technique focuses on realigning deep layers of muscles and connective tissues, addressing persistent pains and stiffness in the neck, lower back, and legs. By applying concentrated pressure using slow, deep strokes, this massage helps physically break down muscle "knots" or adhesions that can disrupt circulation and cause pain, limited range of motion, and inflammation.

Integrating massage therapy into your overall care plan during menopause can provide cumulative benefits, helping to maintain reduced stress levels, pain relief, and sustained mood improvement. Consider scheduling a massage session bi-weekly or monthly beneficial, especially when timed to coincide with peaks in stress or discomfort. This consistency not only aids in maintaining the therapeutic benefits but also offers something to look forward to as a form of self-care and personal nurturing.

Look for a certified massage therapist trained to understand the body's physiology, including changes during menopause. When searching for a therapist, consider asking about their qualifications, experience, and any additional training in techniques beneficial for menopausal symptoms. A good therapist will also create a tailored approach to address your specific needs, adjusting pressure and focus areas as required. They should provide a comfortable, respectful environment where you feel safe and relaxed, allowing for the most beneficial experience.

Massage therapy is more than just a relaxation method; it is a multifaceted therapy that can address the physical and emotional aspects of your transition through menopause. Embrace the healing power of touch as a natural adjunct to other therapies you might be using to enhance your overall strategy for managing menopause with grace and ease.

This chapter has explored various natural and alternative therapies, including herbal remedies, acupuncture, aromatherapy, and massage therapy, as valuable tools for managing menopause. Each modality offers unique benefits, from balancing hormones and reducing symptoms to improving emotional well-being and physical health. As you consider these options, consider them complementary tools, enhancing the other and creating a personalized approach to menopause management.

∽

SELF-CARE AND EMPOWERMENT

*N*avigating menopause can feel like standing at a crossroads where each path represents different facets of your life—personal, professional, and social. As you transition through this phase, these paths might seem more intertwined than ever, with each step affected by your physical and emotional state. During this time, self-care becomes a crucial strategy for maintaining your well-being. In this chapter, we explore how setting boundaries is not only an act of self-preservation but also an expression of self-respect. It involves recognizing your needs, communicating them clearly, and maintaining a balance that keeps you at your best.

SETTING BOUNDARIES: MENTALLY, PHYSICALLY, AND EMOTIONALLY

Self-care is often pictured as indulging in a hot bath or treating yourself to a spa day. While these are delightful aspects of caring for oneself, true self-care during menopause involves deeper, more fundamental practices. It's about setting boundaries that protect and nurture your physical, emotional, and social health. This approach ensures that your energy is focused on activities that nourish rather than deplete you.

Menopause can significantly alter your physical and emotional landscape, making it essential to reassess your needs. What worked for you in the past might no longer work. Physical needs might now include more time for rest or altered dietary requirements, while emotional needs might encompass seeking support or needing more personal space. Socially, your tolerance for engagements may shift. To identify these needs, engage in regular check-ins with yourself. Reflect on what makes you feel balanced and fulfilled versus what leaves you feeling drained.

Communicating Needs

Once you have identified your needs, the next step is to communicate them effectively to those around you—family, friends, or colleagues. Communication should be clear, calm, and assertive. For example, if you need more alone time to recharge, you might say, "I value our time together, but I need a bit more quiet time to feel my best. Let's plan our gatherings at a time when I can be fully present." This approach sets your boundaries while considering the feelings of others.

Recognizing Limits

Menopause might affect your stamina, emotional resilience, and mental clarity. You can set boundaries proactively rather than reactively. This might mean saying no to additional responsibilities before they become a burden or scaling back on commitments that no longer align with your energy levels. Recognizing and respecting your limits is a crucial aspect of self-care that helps prevent burnout.

Boundary-Setting Techniques

Setting boundaries is a skill that can be honed through techniques such as:

> **Scheduled Downtime**: Block time in your calendar for rest and activities that rejuvenate you, making these appointments non-negotiable.
> **Prepared Responses**: Prepare responses for requests or

invitations that might infringe on your boundaries—such as, "Let me check my schedule and get back to you," which gives you time to decide without feeling pressured.

Communicating Boundaries

Practical boundary setting is complemented by effective communication. Use "I" statements to express how certain actions affect you, keeping the focus on your feelings rather than blaming others. For instance, "I feel overwhelmed when I have back-to-back meetings. Could we space them out a bit more?"

Dealing with Pushback

When you assert your boundaries, pushback can sometimes occur. It's essential to stand firm, reiterating your needs calmly and clearly. Setting boundaries is not about being confrontational. Instead, it is about maintaining your well-being. If resistance persists, reaffirm your boundaries with additional explanations: "I understand this may be disappointing, but for me to be fully engaged and healthy, I need to stick to this decision."

In setting boundaries during menopause, you're not creating barriers but defining your space where personal growth and well-being can thrive. This practice benefits you and sets a powerful example for those around you, demonstrating the importance of self-respect and care through all of life's transitions. As you implement these strategies, you empower yourself to navigate menopause not as a time of loss but as one rich with potential for personal growth and discovery.

THE ART OF SELF-COMPASSION DURING MENOPAUSE

Self-compassion might seem gentle, but it's a powerful and necessary practice during the transformative period of menopause. Understanding self-compassion involves recognizing that being kind to yourself is not a luxury but a necessity. It means treating yourself with the same kindness, concern, and support you would offer a good friend. During menopause, your body and emotions undergo significant changes, making it easy to be harsh on yourself during moments of frustration or discomfort. Self-compassion shifts this narrative, helping you to embrace these changes with understanding and patience rather than judgment or self-criticism.

Practicing mindfulness is a foundational aspect of cultivating self-compassion. It involves staying present and engaging fully with the here and now without over-identifying with your thoughts or emotions. For example, during a hot flash or an unexpected wave of emotion, instead of succumbing to negative self-talk like "I can't handle this" or "Something must be wrong with me," mindfulness encourages you to observe these experiences without judgment. By acknowledging your thoughts and feelings with curiosity rather than criticism, you create a space of calmness around them, reducing their intensity and your distress.

To weave self-compassion into your daily life, consider integrating specific practices that foster this mindset.

> **Journaling:** Track and reflect on your experiences with kindness. Each evening, you might write about moments when you felt overwhelmed or critical toward yourself and reframe these incidents more compassionately. For example, if you're frustrated with your forgetfulness, you might write, "It's understandable to forget things when you're going through so much. It's okay to be imperfect."
> **Affirmations:** Use self-kindness affirmations to strengthen your compassionate voice. Phrases such as "I'm doing the best I can," "I am worthy of care," and "I accept myself as I am" can be powerful reminders, especially during tough times.

Menopause also often brings with it societal pressures that can distort your self-image. There is a pervasive cultural narrative that devalues aging, particularly for women, by glorifying youth as the standard of beauty and worth. This societal backdrop can make navigating menopause even more challenging, as it might feel like an erasure of identity or a diminishing of self-worth. Actively rejecting these societal norms and redefining what beauty, strength, and vitality mean to you is crucial. Surround yourself with positive influences—people who celebrate their age, books that discuss menopause openly and positively, or social media accounts that advocate for age positivity. By curating your environment in such a way, you reinforce the notion that menopause is not a decline but another stage of growth and evolution, rich with opportunities for self-discovery and renewal.

Embracing self-compassion during menopause is an empowering act. It allows you to navigate this transition with grace and kindness. Through mindfulness, journaling, affirmations, and challenging societal stereotypes, you can manage menopause symptoms more effectively and enhance your overall well-being. This approach not only transforms how you experience menopause but also sets a profound example for others in your life, spreading the powerful message that self-compassion is an essential part of living fully and aging beautifully.

DIGITAL HEALTH: APPS AND ONLINE RESOURCES FOR MENOPAUSE MANAGEMENT

In today's tech-driven world, digital tools and resources offer valuable support for managing menopause. Engaging with apps designed specifically for menopause can provide insights into your health trends, helping you track symptoms, monitor triggers, and even predict flare-ups. These apps often include features such as symptom trackers, personalized health insights, and daily wellness tips tailored to your unique health profile. For example, some apps allow you to track symptoms and offer educational content on menopause, helping you connect the dots between your lifestyle choices and symptom patterns. This information empowers you to make informed decisions about your health and lifestyle modifications.

The value of online communities during menopause cannot be overstated. Platforms like Menopause Matters Forum or the Reddit Menopause community offer spaces where you can share experiences, seek advice, and find solidarity with others navigating similar challenges. These forums can be incredibly validating and combat the isolation that often accompanies menopause. They allow you to engage in conversations ranging from the best natural remedies for hot flashes to advice on handling emotional changes, offering a comprehensive peer support system. Many of these communities are moderated by health professionals who provide expert insights and debunk myths, ensuring that the information shared is both supportive and scientifically sound.

Telehealth services have revolutionized how we access healthcare, which is particularly advantageous during menopause. Online consultations with healthcare providers who specialize in menopause can be a game-changer, especially for those living in areas with limited access to specialized care. These services offer greater flexibility and privacy, removing the need for travel and waiting rooms. Providers can prescribe medications, recommend lifestyle changes, and provide therapeutic support, all within a virtual setting. This can be particularly helpful for discussing sensitive issues such as sexual health or mental health struggles, which you might find difficult to address in a traditional healthcare setting.

Accessing reliable, evidence-based information on menopause health online is crucial in an age of misinformation. Websites such as The Menopause Society (menopause.org) provide a treasure trove of resources vetted by health professionals. These resources include detailed articles, research updates, and guidelines on topics ranging from hormonal changes to the latest treatment options. Learning to discern credible sources involves checking the authors' credentials, the sources' citations, and the information's transparency. Look for sites that regularly update their content and reference scientific research to ensure you receive the most current and reliable information.

By embracing these digital tools and resources, you are integrating a powerful ally into your menopause management strategy. These resources can offer personalized support, expert advice, community connection, and a wealth of information, all at your fingertips.

Whether tracking health, connecting with others, consulting with specialists, or educating yourself, the digital landscape provides a multifaceted support system that empowers you to take control of your menopause journey with confidence and informed clarity.

ADVOCATING FOR YOUR HEALTH: NAVIGATING THE HEALTHCARE SYSTEM

Menopause symptoms can ebb and flow unpredictably, often feeling overwhelming, so being well-informed is your first line of defense. Understanding various treatment options available isn't just about filling your mind with facts—it's about equipping yourself with the knowledge to make decisions that best suit your unique body and lifestyle. Each piece of information you gather becomes part of your wellness toolkit; the more tools you have, the better prepared you are to navigate menopause.

Start by investing time in learning about the biological processes of menopause. Look for reputable books, websites, and medical journals for the latest research and treatments. Knowing the basics of how hormone levels fluctuate and the potential impacts on your body can transform a conversation with your healthcare provider from a passive appointment into an active dialogue where you're deeply engaged in crafting your care plan.

Effective communication with healthcare providers is key. Approach each appointment as a collaboration, a meeting of experts where you are the expert on your body and experiences, and your provider brings their medical expertise. Prepare for appointments by writing down your symptoms, noting their frequency and severity, and listing any questions or concerns you have. This preparation ensures you make the most of your appointment time with your healthcare provider. Be clear and assertive about your symptoms and concerns, and don't hesitate to express reservations about any recommended treatment that doesn't sit right with you. It's also helpful to repeat what you understand from the conversation to ensure there's no miscommunication. Remember, a good healthcare provider appreciates informed patients who actively participate in their health decisions.

There are moments in healthcare, particularly during complex conditions such as menopause, where a second opinion is a crucial step for you. If a diagnosis doesn't feel quite right or a treatment plan seems off-track, getting another opinion is a proactive step that can provide reassurance or offer new options. It's important to remember that seeking a second opinion is a common practice and is generally supported by healthcare professionals who understand that complex health issues can benefit from multiple expert perspectives. When doing so, choose a specialist in menopause-related issues and take along our medical records and a list of previous treatments. This information can provide a comprehensive view of your health journey and help the consulting physician offer a fresh perspective that is more aligned with your needs.

Navigating the healthcare system requires more than just showing up to appointments. Utilizing healthcare navigation tools can demystify the process, providing guidance such as finding the right specialist to understanding complex medical bills. Health insurance providers often offer resources such as patient advocates or care navigators who can assist with coordinating care, choosing providers, and resolving issues with insurance claims. Online platforms can help you compare healthcare providers, book appointments, and review treatment options. These resources simplify your healthcare logistics, allowing you to focus more on your health and less on the bureaucracy of the healthcare system.

By embracing these strategies—educating yourself, communicating effectively, seeking second opinions, and utilizing navigation tools—you not only ensure that you receive the care you need but also foster a sense of support that can make navigating this transition smoother and more positive. Each step you take empowers you to navigate this transition with confidence and clarity.

MINDSET SHIFTS: VIEWING MENOPAUSE AS A NEW BEGINNING

Menopause is often shrouded in misconceptions and dread, portrayed as a definitive end to youth and vitality. However, what if we reframe this narrative and view menopause not as an ending but as a promising new beginning? This shift in perspective is more than positive thinking; it's about recognizing and embracing the profound transformation that menopause represents. It's a time ripe for personal growth and redefining identity and aspirations.

Reframing menopause begins by dismantling the negative stereotypes that society often perpetuates. Rather than viewing it as a series of physical and emotional challenges to be endured, see it as a significant life transition filled with opportunities. Like any major life shift, menopause allows a chance to pause, reflect, and redirect. It's a perfect time to take inventory of your life's desires and ambitions. What dreams or goals were set aside due to career demands, family care, or lack of time? This phase of life might prompt you to rekindle those aspirations or discover new passions. Embrace menopause as a liberating shift—freeing up energy previously directed toward others to focus on yourself.

Celebrating the wisdom you've accumulated over the years is invaluable. Menopause marks a milestone that underscores this wealth of wisdom and highlights your hard-earned experiences, knowledge, and insights. It's a time to acknowledge and leverage this intellectual and emotional capital. Reflecting on the challenges you've overcome and the magnitude of the understanding you've gained. This wisdom is a powerful tool, not just for personal growth, but it can also inspire and guide others. Sharing your journey and insights can support other women, creating a community that values and respects the wisdom that comes with age.

Looking forward, menopause can be a springboard into a fulfilling new phase of life. With changing family dynamics or reduced career pressures shifting, you may find more time to focus on personal development and self-care. Use this period to set new health goals, travel to places you've always wanted to visit or dive deeper into hobbies that bring you joy. Recognize the potential of menopause as a time to embrace new opportunities rather than focusing on what's being left behind.

Education plays a pivotal role in making menopause a positive experience. Understanding the physiological changes and how they affect your body demystifies the process and reduces anxiety. Educating yourself about nutritional needs, physical health strategies, and emotional wellness during menopause empowers you with the tools to manage symptoms effectively and maintain your quality of life. Moreover, engaging in continuous learning — whether through courses, workshops, or even returning to school can invigorate the mind and spirit. This continuous learning transforms menopause into an ongoing journey of growth and discovery.

By adopting these mindset shifts, menopause becomes more than just an end to fertility—it transforms into a celebration of maturity and a renaissance of self. As you adapt to these changes, remember menopause is not merely a phase to manage but a transition to welcome with open arms and a hopeful heart.

CREATING YOUR MENOPAUSE PLAN: A STEP-BY-STEP GUIDE

Navigating menopause effectively requires a personalized approach. Each woman experiences menopause differently, influenced by individual health backgrounds, lifestyles, and preferences. Creating a customized menopause management plan will serve as your roadmap, guiding you through symptom management, integrating beneficial lifestyle changes, and continuously adapting to your body's evolving needs.

Begin by thoroughly understanding your symptoms and how they impact your daily life. Track your symptoms in detail, noting their frequency, intensity, and triggers. For example, if caffeine late in the day disrupts your sleep or spicy foods seem to increase hot flashes, this level of detail can help identify patterns and pinpoint which lifestyle adjustments yield the most significant benefits. With this information, you can work with healthcare providers to develop a symptom management strategy that addresses your most pressing concerns. This strategy might include a combination of dietary adjustments, prescribed medications, or even alternative therapies such as acupuncture or yoga, depending on what best aligns with your symptoms and personal health philosophy.

Incorporate lifestyle changes gradually into your daily routine. These adjustments should enhance your quality of life without overwhelming you. For sleep disruptions, establish a calming bedtime routine—dim the lights an hour before bed, disconnect from digital devices, and perhaps engage in relaxing activities like reading or meditation. For dietary changes, gradually add phytoestrogen-rich foods such as flaxseed and soy products to your meals to help balance hormone levels. Consistency is vital to making these changes part of your daily life.

Monitoring progress is a process that requires regular reassessment and adaptation. As you adapt and your body changes, your responses to treatments can also change. Set regular intervals—every three to six months, for example—to review the effectiveness of your menopause plan. Revisit your symptom journal, evaluate the impact of lifestyle changes, and discuss these with your healthcare provider. Such reviews help identify what's working and what needs adjustment. For instance, if certain supplements or exercises lose effectiveness, it may be time to explore new options. Keeping an open dialogue with your healthcare provider ensures your plan stays current.

Adjust your plan as needed. As you monitor your progress, you may discover an activity or food that unexpectedly affects your symptoms. If emotional symptoms become more pronounced, for example, consider incorporating additional psychological support or stress management strategies. Adjusting your plan as your symptoms evolve ensures effective management. Remaining flexible and responsive to these changes is crucial in controlling your menopause experience.

Adjusting your plan as needed is a natural part of the process. As you monitor your progress, you'll gain insights that may prompt changes to your management strategy. Perhaps a new symptom emerges, or you discover an activity or food that unexpectedly affects your symptoms. Adjustments might also include shifting the focus of your plan as your symptoms evolve. For instance, if emotional symptoms become more pronounced over time, your plan might move to include more psychological support or stress management strategies. Remaining flexible and responsive to these changes is crucial in controlling your menopause experience.

By crafting a personalized menopause plan, you empower yourself to navigate this transition proactively. Understanding your unique symptoms, integrating lifestyle changes, monitoring progress, and adapting your strategy creates a dynamic framework supporting your health and well-being. This tailored approach enhances symptom management and enriches your quality of life during this significant phase.

In this chapter, we've outlined a comprehensive, adaptable blueprint for managing menopause. Emphasizing a personalized approach, developing detailed symptom management strategies, and adjusting your lifestyle as needed constitute a plan designed to evolve with you. Remember that this menopause plan is not static; it is an ongoing process of adaptation and growth.

MOVING FORWARD WITH CONFIDENCE

*A*s the sun sets on the horizon of menopause, a new dawn emerges, revealing a landscape rich with potential and promise. This phase of your life, postmenopause, is about thriving with newfound wisdom and experiences. Embrace it as a time of revitalization, where each day holds the potential for growth and joy.

LIFE AFTER MENOPAUSE: WHAT TO EXPECT

In postmenopause, many women find that their symptoms begin to stabilize, offering a welcomed reprieve. However, the journey toward maintaining your physical health should not pause. On the contrary, this is the perfect time to reinforce your commitment to a healthy lifestyle. Regular physical activity remains a cornerstone of good health, helping to maintain muscle mass, manage weight, and reduce the risk of chronic diseases such as diabetes and heart disease. Incorporating strength training into your exercise routine can combat the loss of bone density and muscle mass—a common after menopause. Additionally, staying vigilant about your cardiovascular health through aerobic exercises is vital for keeping your heart strong and your body agile.

Consider integrating activities that align with your natural rhythm and interests. If yoga you brought solace during menopause, perhaps deepen that practice. If walking was your preferred activity, explore new trails or join a walking group that aligns with your pace and interests. The key is to continue activities that you enjoy and are sustainable, fostering a routine that supports your physical health without feeling burdensome.

Emotional and Mental Wellbeing

Postmenopause often brings a greater sense of emotional stability compared to the rollercoaster of perimenopause, allowing you to rediscover your emotional landscape without the intense hormonal changes. It's a time to reconnect with yourself and cultivate inner peace. Meditation, mindfulness, and deep-breathing exercises can enhance your emotional well-being, helping you maintain a calm and centered outlook.

Reflecting on your emotional journey through menopause can be empowering. Recognizing your strength and resilience provides a solid foundation for facing future challenges with grace and confidence. Engaging in social activities that foster positive relationships can enrich your emotional health, offering support and companionship as you navigate this new chapter.

Lifestyle Adjustments

As you move forward, lifestyle adjustments focusing on long-term health and vitality become crucial. Nutrition plays a pivotal role—emphasize heart-healthy diets rich in fruits, vegetables, whole grains, and lean proteins. Considering the metabolic changes postmenopause, a mindful approach to eating can help manage weight and promote overall health. Moreover, ensuring adequate calcium and vitamin D intake supports bone health, which is especially important as you age.

Sleep, often disrupted during menopause, may improve as hormone levels stabilize. Good sleep hygiene practices can enhance sleep quality and positively impact overall health, including mental clarity and energy levels throughout the day.

The New Normal

Embracing postmenopause as your new normal involves acknowledging and accepting the changes that have occurred. It's about building on the adjustments you've made and viewing them not as temporary fixes but as permanent improvements to your lifestyle. Acceptance allows you to live fully, embracing the changes menopause has brought with confidence and positivity. It's also a time to celebrate the freedom that comes with this phase—freedom from menstrual cycles and the unpredictability of perimenopause. Now, you can focus on what brings joy and fulfillment, exploring new interests and deepening existing passions.

Remember that moving forward confidently isn't about erasing the past but building on the experiences and knowledge you've gained. Step into your post-menopausal life with hope and a proactive plan that celebrates and supports your ongoing journey of health and happiness.

PREVENTIVE HEALTH: STAYING AHEAD OF AGE-RELATED CONCERNS

Navigating your post-menopausal years with finesse involves a proactive stance on preventive health. Regular health screenings are crucial checkpoints, helping you stay informed about your body's condition and catching potential issues before they escalate. Bone density tests are essential for assessing bone strength, given the increased risk of osteoporosis due to lower estrogen levels. Cardiovascular health also requires close monitoring, as heart disease risk tends to rise after menopause. Regular check-ups, including blood pressure monitoring and cholesterol checks, are essential to your health regimen.

A balanced, nutrient-rich diet is pivotal in staving off age-related health issues. Your diet should be rich in calcium and vitamin D to support bone health, while foods high in omega-3 fatty acids can benefit your heart health. Antioxidant-rich foods, such as berries and leafy greens, combat inflammation and support overall cellular health. Staying hydrated is essential as it impacts everything from your skin to the functionality of your kidneys. Adjustments in your diet can have profound effects not only on your physical health but also on your overall vitality, aiding in everything from improved energy levels to better cognitive function.

Cognitive health often becomes a concern as one ages, with worries about memory decline or decreased mental agility. Engage your brain in activities that challenge and stimulate cognitive functions, such as puzzles, learning a new language, or even playing musical instruments. Social engagement is also crucial for maintaining cognitive health. Regular interactions with friends, family, and community can help keep your mind sharp and alert. Lifelong learning, whether through formal education or personal hobbies, stimulates neural pathways and enriches daily life.

Embracing holistic health practices offers a comprehensive approach to wellness that aligns with your physical, mental, and emotional health. Yoga and tai chi promote physical flexibility and strength while contributing to mental clarity and stress reduction. Meditation provides a sanctuary of calm, helping you to manage stress effectively and supporting overall health. These practices create a balanced approach to health that keeps you thriving.

REINVENTING SEXUALITY AND INTIMACY IN LATER LIFE

The post-menopausal years often bring profound transformations in how you experience and express intimacy and sexuality. Freed from the reproductive concerns, this period invites a deeper exploration of what intimacy means to you now. Your capacity for rich, fulfilling relationships can expand, offering new dimensions of closeness.

You might notice a shift in the dynamics of your relationships. This is a time to communicate openly with your partner about your desires and explore new ways to connect that may have been overlooked in earlier years. For some, this may mean exploring new levels of emotional intimacy by sharing thoughts and experiences more openly. For others, it might involve trying new activities together, such as dance classes or travel, transforming shared experiences into deeper bonds.

The evolution of intimacy also involves reconnecting with your body's new state. Menopause can change your physical responses and needs, making candid conversations about sexual health with your partner crucial. Discussing what feels different, what feels good, and where you may need support or adjustments enhances mutual understanding and ensures that physical intimacy remains a source of joy and comfort.

Addressing the physical aspects of post-menopausal sexuality is equally important. Changes such as decreased natural lubrication can be approached with practical solutions like the use of water-based lubricants or moisturizers, significantly enhancing comfort during intercourse. Additionally, engaging in regular pelvic floor exercises can improve both physical health and sexual function. These exercises strengthen the pelvic muscles, which can enhance sensation and sexual satisfaction while also helping to prevent or manage urinary incontinence, a common issue after menopause.

This phase of your life offers a unique opportunity to redefine and deepen your understanding of intimacy and sexuality. By embracing open communication, fostering emotional connections, exploring personal desires, and addressing physical changes with practical solutions, you can enjoy a rich and fulfilling sexual life in your postmenopausal years.

THE IMPORTANCE OF COMMUNITY AND SOCIAL CONNECTIONS

Building and nurturing a support network can remarkably transform your post-menopausal experience into a vibrant season of connection and mutual growth. As you adjust to the new rhythms of your life, surrounding yourself in a community that uplifts and supports you becomes essential. This network isn't just about having people around; it's about cultivating relationships that provide emotional solace, social engagement, and practical support when needed.

Actively engaging in community activities can help to overcome the sense of isolation that sometimes accompanies menopause. Whether through volunteer work, joining clubs or groups based on personal interests, or participating in local events, each interaction weaves you deeper into the social fabric. These activities enrich your daily life and anchor you in a community that offers diverse perspectives and support. For example, joining a gardening club nurtures your hobby while connecting you with like-minded individuals who can share in your challenges and victories, both inside and outside the garden.

The richness of inter-generational relationships is particularly profound during this stage of life. These connections weave a tapestry of wisdom, energy, and new perspectives that can enhance your understanding and enjoyment of the world. The wisdom shared by older generations can offer a long-view perspective that enriches your life's narrative. Younger people provide fresh insights and vitality and can challenge you to view the world differently. This mutually beneficial exchange fosters a sense of continuity and legacy that bolsters everyone involved. Engaging with various generations, whether within your family, community, or even through mentorship programs, can be incredibly rewarding.

Leveraging Online Communities

In today's digital era, online platforms and social media offer unprecedented opportunities for connecting with others across the globe who share your interests and experiences. For women navigating postmenopause, online communities can be a goldmine of resources, support, and camaraderie. These platforms enable you to share stories, exchange tips and offer encouragement without the constraints of geography. They can be particularly helpful for those living in remote areas or with mobility constraints.

Engaging with virtual communities goes beyond passive scrolling; it means actively participating in discussions, sharing your experiences, and offering a listening ear to others. Many find that these interactions lead to friendships as real and meaningful as those formed in person. Moreover, the anonymity and accessibility of online platforms can sometimes make it easier to discuss sensitive topics, such as sexual health or emotional struggles, which you might find difficult to address face-to-face.

A NEW CHAPTER: MENOPAUSE AS A GATEWAY TO REDISCOVERING YOURSELF

Menopause, often seen as an ending, can hold the seeds of new beginnings. This pivotal phase invites you to rediscover who you are. It beckons you to explore personal growth, self-reflection, and a renewed focus on passions that may have been sidelined in the bustling years of earlier adulthood. Engage in self-reflection as a review of the past and a forward-looking exploration to understand how your desires and aspirations have evolved. This reflective practice can uncover aspects of your character and desires that were overshadowed by the demands of earlier life stages.

Embracing the changes brought on by menopause requires an open-minded approach to your body and mind's transformations. While these changes can be challenging, they also open doors to new opportunities. Shifts in hormonal levels may alter how you experience and interact with the world around you. This new perspective can inspire a reevaluation of what truly matters to you. Perhaps you discover a burgeoning interest in environmental issues or a dormant desire to try pottery. Embracing these changes as opportunities enriches your life and personal identity.

Reevaluating your priorities becomes not just necessary but exciting. It allows you to align your daily actions with your interests and values. This could mean scaling back on professional responsibilities to make room for volunteering or prioritizing travel and cultural exploration over previous routines that no longer bring joy. Consider what genuinely brings you satisfaction and fulfillment. This process isn't about making abrupt changes but about gradually aligning your life with your evolving self, ensuring that each day is lived following your deepest values and joys.

Self-expression during this time becomes a vital outlet and a powerful form of exploration. Whether through creative endeavors such as writing and painting or public expressions such as advocacy or community leadership, these outlets allow you to share your unique perspective and experiences. Starting a blog, joining a local writing group, or taking art classes are not just hobbies but expressions of your inner self. Each action weaves a thread into the larger tapestry of who you are becoming in this postmenopausal phase.

Exploring new interests or rekindling old passions can be incredibly rejuvenating. Menopause often provides the time and impetus to revisit long-held interests, whether that's enrolling in a dance class, learning a new language, or picking up a musical instrument. These activities enrich your life, offering new challenges and joys that counteract feelings of stagnation or isolation.

Lifelong learning plays a vital role in this new phase. It keeps the mind sharp and the spirit engaged. Learning is a lifelong journey, and continuing to educate yourself can be one of the most rewarding ways to spend your post-menopausal years. Whether through formal education, such as enrolling in university courses, or less formal means, such as attending workshops or listening to webinars, every bit of new knowledge enriches your understanding of the world and your place in it.

Setting new goals or revisiting old ones can give a renewed sense of purpose and direction. Postmenopause, with its shift in responsibilities and changes in personal identity, offers a unique opportunity to set goals that resonate with who you are now. These goals should not only aim to achieve outward successes but should also foster personal satisfaction and growth. They might involve physical fitness, mastering a new skill, or achieving a long-held dream. These goals provide motivation and make your postmenopausal years something not just to survive but to enjoy.

EMBRACING AGING WITH GRACE AND STRENGTH

Societal narratives often cast aging in a negative light, especially for women. It becomes important to illuminate the positive aspects, celebrating each year as a testament to your journey and wisdom.

Embrace aging as a natural and enriching process frames age as an emblem of life's well-lived chapters rather than merely the passage of time.

Challenging ageist stereotypes begins with changing the internal dialogue about aging. Society often glorifies youth while marginalizing the older populations, particularly postmenopausal women. Confront these stereotypes head-on, questioning their validity, and reframing aging as a period rich with opportunities for continued growth and exploration. Embrace your age with pride! Every wrinkle tells a story of laughter, and every gray hair highlights your life's journey. By adopting this mindset, you empower yourself and challenge societal norms that define beauty and worth by age.

Focusing on wellness practices that promote vitality and health at any age is crucial in maintaining your zest for life. Engage in activities that nourish both the body and soul—through regular physical exercise that keeps your body strong and limber or through hobbies that ignite your spirit. Balanced nutrition and adequate sleep support your physical health. Remember, wellness extends beyond the physical and encompasses mental and emotional health. Engage in practices that reduce stress and enhance your emotional equilibrium, such as mindfulness or connecting with nature, which profoundly affect overall well-being.

This period of your life is an opportunity to redefine beauty standards. The beauty industry often overlooks the older demographic, with most products targeted at anti-aging, suggesting that aging is something to be hidden rather than embraced. It's time to shift this narrative. Support brands that celebrate age-inclusive beauty, highlight the natural aging process, and showcase diverse ages in their campaigns. By choosing products and practices that honor aging, you foster self-acceptance and love and reinforce the idea that beauty transcends age.

Highlighting role models who exemplify aging with grace and strength can be incredibly inspiring. Look to people in various fields—arts, politics, science, or your community—who confidently embrace their age and continue to make significant contributions.

These role models shatter stereotypes and demonstrate that aging can be a dynamic and positive experience filled with continued achievements and adventures. Draw inspiration from their stories. Their journeys motivate you to pursue your passions with renewed vigor, regardless of age.

Embracing aging with grace and strength, you redefine what it means to grow older. It's about celebrating the journey thus far while looking forward to each new year's opportunities. Age becomes not a countdown but a count-up of experiences, learnings, and joys yet to be discovered. Treat each year as a new chapter, not in the twilight of life but an ongoing saga of growth and fulfillment. This approach enriches your life and challenges the cultural narratives surrounding aging, paving the way for a society that respects and values age in all its complexity.

LEGACY BUILDING: WHAT WILL YOU CREATE NEXT?

As you navigate the serene waters of postmenopause, consider the impact of your life's journey. Legacy is often thought of in terms of grand achievements or substantial gifts. Yet, the true essence lies in everyday interactions, choices, and passions. It's about the mark you leave on the world—tangible and intangible—and how it ripples through generations. Reflect on the values and lessons that have been significant in your life. How can these be shared or passed on?

Creating a family legacy could involve compiling family stories, recipes, and traditions into a book that can be passed down. It can also be about embedding values like kindness, resilience, and curiosity into the fabric of family life. Beyond family, your career and other interests offer platforms for influence. Consider mentoring younger colleagues or setting up a scholarship to support those starting their journey. Each of these acts extends your impact, planting seeds for future growth.

Your influence can also extend into the broader community. Engaging in volunteer work not only addresses immediate needs but also sets a precedent for civic responsibility. Whether helping beautify local parks, participating in community education programs, or supporting local art initiatives, community service enriches both the giver and the receiver. It's about crafting a legacy of care and engagement that strengthens the community's health for years to come.

Creative endeavors provide another profound medium for legacy building. Whether you paint, write, craft, or perform, your creative works can reflect your inner world and inspire, challenge, and comfort others long after they are made, serving as lasting testaments to your vision and spirit.

Documenting your life stories, wisdom, and experiences is also vital to legacy building. Consider writing a memoir, starting a blog, or recording video messages. These narratives can connect and guide future generations, helping them navigate their paths with your wisdom.

Mentorship extends the legacy of your professional and personal life by weaving your experiences, insights, and guidance into the growth trajectories of others. Serving as a mentor enables you to give back in a deeply personal way, helping mentees through challenges you've navigated, sharing mistakes and successes, and helping them forge their paths. It's a profound way to ensure that your hard-earned wisdom reverberates through time.

Remember that the most enduring legacies are those that make a positive impact on others' lives. They are crafted through consistent actions, choices, and commitments that reflect who you are. Think about the values you wish to champion and the memories you want to leave behind. Whether through family, work, community, or creative expression, your legacy reflects your life's work and love—a lasting imprint that inspires and influences future generations.

THE MENOPAUSE MOVEMENT: BECOMING PART OF THE CHANGE AND EMPOWER THE NEXT GENERATION

In the quiet moments of reflection after the menopause storm, many women find themselves poised to use their experiences as catalysts for change. This newfound perspective offers a chance for broader societal impact. The Menopause Movement aims to shift the narrative from silence and stigma to openness and empowerment. By engaging in this movement, you can help shape a more informed and inclusive society that supports women through all stages of life.

Breaking the Silence

Encouraging open dialogue about menopause is the first step toward dismantling the taboos surrounding this natural life stage. For too long, women have navigated menopause quietly, often feeling isolated due to a lack of open conversation. By speaking openly about your journey, you contribute to a culture of transparency that can liberate others. Consider starting or joining discussion groups, whether in person or online, where menopause is the main topic. Please share your story, the challenges you faced, how you overcame them, and the lessons learned. These narratives are powerful; they validate personal experiences and build bridges of empathy and understanding within families, friendships, and even with healthcare providers.

Advocacy and Awareness

As you grow more comfortable sharing your story, use your voice for advocacy, pushing for greater menopause awareness, education, and research. Many women are underprepared for menopause due to a lack of accessible information. By advocating for menopause education in public health discussions, pushing for research on menopausal health, or lobbying for better training for healthcare providers, you help ensure that future generations of women are better equipped to manage menopause. Participation in health forums, community outreach programs, or even online platforms can amplify your advocacy efforts, turning personal passion into public benefit.

Creating Supportive Spaces

Building spaces that support menopausal awareness and education can significantly impact community health. If you are part of a workplace, advocate for policies that help menopausal women, such as flexible work hours or environments sensitive to menopausal symptoms like temperature fluctuations. In community settings, consider facilitating or supporting workshops that educate women on menopause management strategies or holistic health approaches. These initiatives aid in personal health management and foster community solidarity and support, making menopause a shared topic rather than a private struggle.

Policy and Workplace Change

In the broader socio-economic sphere, there is a pressing need for policies that recognize and accommodate the unique needs of menopausal women. This involves advocating for workplace policies that include menopausal symptoms, such as providing more flexible sick leave policies or wellness programs that address specific menopausal concerns. By engaging with human resources professionals, sharing insightful articles, or even organizing informational sessions with healthcare professionals, you can influence policy changes that make the daily realities of working menopausal women more manageable.

Global Perspectives

Engaging with the global menopause movement can enrich your understanding and approach to menopause management. Different cultures offer varying insights into menopause management that can be adapted or adopted.

Participating in international forums, following global health organizations, or simply connecting with women online from diverse backgrounds can broaden your perspective. This global exchange of ideas fosters a worldwide support network that transcends cultural and geographical boundaries.

By contributing to the Menopause Movement, you help shift the narrative toward greater awareness, support, and empowerment for all women experiencing menopause. This engagement transforms personal experiences into public advocacy and ensures that the journey through menopause is recognized and respected worldwide as an important aspect of women's health. Through dialogue, advocacy, and community engagement, you help pave the way for a society that embraces and supports women throughout all phases of life, ensuring that the legacy of today's efforts will benefit the health and well-being of future generations.

From breaking the silence and advocating for comprehensive education to creating supportive environments and embracing a global perspective, your involvement in the Menopause Movement shapes a future where menopause is met with understanding and support.

CONCLUSION

As we wrap up our enriching journey through the book *Master Menopause*, it's time to reflect on the transformative path we've shared. From navigating initial uncertainty and fear to discovering empowerment and control, this book stands as a testament to the profound impact of understanding and embracing menopause. We've ventured beyond the end of menstrual cycles to uncover the emotional, physical, and societal dimensions of this significant life stage.

Menopause encompasses not only physical changes but also mental and emotional shifts. Addressing these mental health challenges that often accompany this period is not optional—it's essential. This book emphasizes the power of understanding, recognizing both physical transformations and their profound emotional and psychological impacts. Remember, knowledge is not just power; it is empowerment. By demystifying the symptoms and processes of menopause, we've equipped you with the tools to navigate this phase with informed confidence and a greater sense of control over your body and mind.

The personal stories and insights shared throughout these chapters validate the individual experiences and weave a rich tapestry of collective wisdom and support. These narratives highlight the importance of inclusivity, reminding us that while each journey is unique, our experiences are interconnected.

We've embraced a holistic approach to managing menopause, covering everything from dietary adjustments and physical exercises to mental health strategies and both traditional and alternative treatments. Each strategy is presented not as a one-size-fits-all solution but as a suggestion for personal adaptation, underscoring the need for a tailored, integrative approach to manage menopause effectively.

Menopause is not an end but a continuing narrative of self-discovery, growth, and fulfillment. It invites us to remain proactive—seeking support, staying informed, and advocating for ourselves and others. The journey does not end here. I urge you to continue educating yourself, join or initiate advocacy efforts for improved menopausal care, and lend your voice to elevate this vital conversation.

I invite you to share your own stories and experiences. By doing so, you contribute to a vibrant, ongoing dialogue that supports and enriches our community. Your insights and experiences are invaluable, and they deserve to be heard. Your unique perspective can inspire and guide others, making you an integral part of this community.

With the insights and strategies you've gained from this book, you can approach menopause with acceptance, confidence, grace, and anticipation. Continue to advocate for your health, seek joy in your experiences, and embrace this significant phase of life with open arms and a hopeful heart.

Thank you for trusting me to be a part of your journey. May you move forward with a fortified spirit and an empowered mind, ready to embrace all of life's richness beyond menopause.

REFERENCES

BASE. (n.d.). Surprising ways meditation changes your stress hormone. https://getbase.com/blog/meditation-hormones

Breastcancer.org. (n.d.). Hormone replacement therapy and breast cancer risk. https://www.breastcancer.org/risk/risk-factors/using-hormone-replacement-therapy

British Dietetic Association (BDA). (n.d.). Menopause and diet. https://www.bda.uk.com/resource/menopause-diet.html

Cleveland Clinic. (n.d.). Perimenopause: Age, stages, signs, symptoms & treatment. https://my.clevelandclinic.org/health/diseases/21608-perimenopause

Endocrine Society. (n.d.). Menopause and bone loss. https://www.endocrine.org/patient-engagement/endocrine-library/menopause-and-bone-loss

Everyday Health. (n.d.). 10 reasons to look forward to menopause. https://www.everydayhealth.com/menopause-pictures/positives-of-menopause.aspx

Harvard Health. (n.d.). Menopause and mental health. https://www.health.harvard.edu/womens-health/menopause-and-mental-health

Harvard Health. (n.d.). Nonhormonal treatments for menopause. https://www.health.harvard.edu/womens-health/nonhormonal-treatments-for-menopause

Healthline. (n.d.). Understanding how your skin changes during menopause. https://www.healthline.com/health/beauty-skin-care/menopause-skin-changes

Hormone Health Network. (n.d.). Menopause support and resources. https://www.endocrine.org/menopausemap/support-resources/index.html

Jefferson Health. (n.d.). The truth about menopause: Debunking 6 common misconceptions. https://www.jeffersonhealth.org/your-health/living-well/the-truth-about-menopause-misconceptions

Johns Hopkins Medicine. (n.d.). How sex changes after menopause. https://www.hopkinsmedicine.org/health/wellness-and-prevention/how-sex-changes-after-menopause

Johns Hopkins Medicine. (n.d.). Introduction to menopause. https://www.hopkinsmedicine.org/health/conditions-and-diseases/introduction-to-menopause

Johns Hopkins Medicine. (n.d.). Staying healthy after menopause. https://www.hopkinsmedicine.org/health/conditions-and-diseases/staying-healthy-after-menopause

Moreland OB/GYN. (n.d.). Yoga for menopause: 8 poses for your symptoms. https://www.morelandobgyn.com/blog/yoga-for-menopause-8-poses-for-your-menopause-symptoms

National Center for Biotechnology Information (NCBI). (n.d.). Efficacy of phytoestrogens for menopausal symptoms. https://www.ncbi.nlm.nih.gov/pmc/articles/PMC4389700/

National Center for Biotechnology Information (NCBI). (n.d.). Exercise beyond menopause: Dos and don'ts. https://www.ncbi.nlm.nih.gov/pmc/articles/PMC3296386/

National Center for Biotechnology Information (NCBI). (n.d.). Hormonal changes during menopause and the impact on ... https://www.ncbi.nlm.nih.gov/pmc/articles/PMC3984489/

National Center for Biotechnology Information (NCBI). (n.d.). How effective the mindfulness-based cognitive behavioral ... https://www.ncbi.nlm.nih.gov/pmc/articles/PMC9583372/

National Center for Biotechnology Information (NCBI). (n.d.). Menopause and the influence of culture: Another gap for ... https://www.ncbi.nlm.nih.gov/pmc/articles/PMC3554544/

National Center for Biotechnology Information (NCBI). (n.d.). Menopause and cognitive impairment: A narrative review ... https://www.ncbi.nlm.nih.gov/pmc/articles/PMC8394691/

National Center for Biotechnology Information (NCBI). (n.d.). Physical activity and exercise for hot flashes: Trigger or ... https://www.ncbi.nlm.nih.gov/pmc/articles/PMC9886316/

National Center for Biotechnology Information (NCBI). (n.d.). Psychosocial factors promoting resilience during the ... https://www.ncbi.nlm.nih.gov/pmc/articles/PMC7979610/

National Institute on Aging (NIA). (n.d.). Hot flashes: What can I do? https://www.nia.nih.gov/health/menopause/hot-flashes-what-can-i-do

National Institutes of Health (NIH). (n.d.). Black cohosh - Health professional fact sheet. https://ods.od.nih.gov/factsheets/BlackCohosh-HealthProfessional/

National Library of Medicine. (n.d.). A comprehensive review of the safety and efficacy ... https://pubmed.ncbi.nlm.nih.gov/17217322/

National Library of Medicine. (n.d.). A double-blinded, randomized placebo controlled clinical trial. https://pubmed.ncbi.nlm.nih.gov/37743153/#:~:text=Conclusion%3A%20The%20study%20found%20that,in%20reducing%20the%20menopausal%20symptoms

National Library of Medicine. (n.d.). Botanical and dietary supplements for menopausal symptoms. https://pubmed.ncbi.nlm.nih.gov/16181020/

NHS Inform. (n.d.). Sexual wellbeing, intimacy and menopause. https://www.nhsinform.scot/healthy-living/womens-health/later-years-around-50-years-and-over/menopause-and-postmenopause-health/sexual-wellbeing-intimacy-and-menopause/

NHS Inform. (n.d.). Supporting someone through the menopause. https://www.nhsinform.scot/healthy-living/womens-health/later-years-around-50-years-and-over/menopause-and-postmenopause-health/supporting-someone-through-the-menopause

NHS. (n.d.). Benefits and risks of hormone replacement therapy (HRT). https://www.nhs.uk/medicines/hormone-replacement-therapy-hrt/benefits-and-risks-of-hormone-replacement-therapy-hrt/

North American Menopause Society (NAMS). (n.d.). Focused on providing physicians, practitioners & women menopause information, help & treatment insights. https://www.menopause.org

North American Menopause Society (NAMS). (n.d.). Staying healthy at menopause and beyond. https://www.menopause.org/for-women/menopauseflashes/women's-health-and-menopause/staying-healthy-at-menopause-and-beyond

NSCA Journal of Strength and Conditioning Research. (2013, October). Maximal strength training in postmenopausal women with ... https://journals.lww.com/nsca-jscr/fulltext/2013/10000/maximal_strength_training_in_postmenopausal_women.32.aspx

Office on Women's Health. (n.d.). Menopause and sexuality. https://www.womenshealth.gov/menopause/menopause-and-sexuality

OSF HealthCare. (n.d.). Navigating menopause: Expert advice for symptom relief. https://newsroom.osfhealthcare.org/navigating-menopause-expert-advice-for-symptom-relief/

Rae, A. (2023, October 18). Beyond hot flashes: A deep dive into menopause, work ... Forbes. https://www.forbes.com/sites/aparnarae/2023/10/18/beyond-hot-flashes-a-deep-dive-into-menopause-work-and-the-economy/

Stella. (n.d.). How to approach finding the positive in menopause. https://www.onstella.com/the-latest/anxiety-and-mood/finding-positivity-in-menopause/

Women's Center of Orlando. (n.d.). 5 self-care tips for thriving through menopause. https://wcorlando.com/5-self-care-tips-for-thriving-through-menopause/

www.ingramcontent.com/pod-product-compliance
Lightning Source LLC
Chambersburg PA
CBHW020548030426
42337CB00013B/1008